THE
EVERYTHING
GLYCEMIC INDEX COOKBOOK
2ND EDITION

Dear Reader,

This book will teach you how to use the glycemic index for meal planning. It includes 300 delicious recipes to keep you well fed with the comfort of knowing you are eating right. No matter what your health goals may be—getting in shape, controlling your appetite, or managing diabetes—this book has a great deal to offer you. You will have the necessary knowledge and tools to use the glycemic index successfully right at your fingertips.

As a registered dietitian (RD), I work with many individuals and families who have struggled with gaining weight, controlling their blood sugar, and balancing their meals. I often hear from my clients that they feel hungry and dissatisfied when dieting. There are many misconceptions about how to eat healthfully. Popular diets are here today and gone the next; however, the glycemic index is here to stay.

A registered dietitian that loves food created the recipes in this book, and they are nutritious without compromising taste. It is important to eat a variety of foods, and the glycemic index allows you to do just this. Put on your chef's hat and get started!

Sincerely,

LeeAnn Smith Weintraub, MPH, RD

Welcome to the EVERYTHING® Series!

These handy, accessible books give you all you need to tackle a difficult project, gain a new hobby, comprehend a fascinating topic, prepare for an exam, or even brush up on something you learned back in school but have since forgotten.

You can choose to read an *Everything®* book from cover to cover or just pick out the information you want from our four useful boxes: e-questions, e-facts, e-alerts, and e-ssentials.

We give you everything you need to know on the subject, but throw in a lot of fun stuff along the way, too.

We now have more than 400 *Everything®* books in print, spanning such wide-ranging categories as weddings, pregnancy, cooking, music instruction, foreign language, crafts, pets, New Age, and so much more. When you're done reading them all, you can finally say you know *Everything®*!

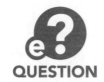

QUESTION
Answers to
common questions

FACT
Important snippets
of information

ALERT
Urgent
warnings

ESSENTIAL
Quick
handy tips

PUBLISHER Karen Cooper

DIRECTOR OF ACQUISITIONS AND INNOVATION Paula Munier

MANAGING EDITOR, EVERYTHING® SERIES Lisa Laing

COPY CHIEF Casey Ebert

ASSISTANT PRODUCTION EDITOR Jacob Erickson

ACQUISITIONS EDITOR Katrina Schroeder

ASSOCIATE DEVELOPMENT EDITOR Hillary Thompson

EDITORIAL ASSISTANT Ross Weisman

EVERYTHING® SERIES COVER DESIGNER Erin Alexander

LAYOUT DESIGNERS Colleen Cunningham, Elisabeth Lariviere, Ashley Vierra, Denise Wallace

Visit the entire Everything® series at *www.everything.com*

THE
EVERYTHING®
GLYCEMIC INDEX
COOKBOOK

2ND EDITION

LeeAnn Smith Weintraub, MPH, RD

Foreword by Ilya Michael Rachman, MD, PhD

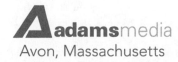

Avon, Massachusetts

I would like to dedicate this book to my husband Matt, who lovingly encourages me to pursue my goals. Thank you for your support, humor, and for believing in me.

An Everything® Series Book.
Everything® and everything.com® are registered trademarks of F+W Media, Inc.

Published by Adams Media, a division of F+W Media, Inc.
57 Littlefield Street, Avon, MA 02322 U.S.A.
www.adamsmedia.com

ISBN 10: 1-4405-0584-5
ISBN 13: 978-1-4405-0584-3
eISBN 10: 1-4405-0585-3
eISBN 13: 978-1-4405-0585-0

Printed in the United States of America.

10 9 8 7 6 5 4

Library of Congress Cataloging-in-Publication Data
The everything® glycemic index cookbook / LeeAnn Smith Weintraub; foreword by Ilya Michael Rachman.
p. cm.
Includes bibliographical references and index.
ISBN 978-1-4405-0584-3 (alk. paper)
1. Low-carbohydrate diet—Recipes. 2. Glycemic index. I. Title.
RM237.73.M33 2010
641.5'6383—dc22
2010027243

This book is available at quantity discounts for bulk purchases.
For information, please call 1-800-289-0963.

Contents

Acknowledgments

I would like to acknowledge those who have helped me in the production process of this book as well as those who have inspired my love of healthy eating. First, thank you to Neil Salkind for introducing me to the world of book publishing. It has been a pleasure working with him on this project. Many thanks to Katrina Schroeder for her assistance and support. I truly appreciate Dr. Ilya Rachman for taking time in his busy schedule to write the foreword.

It is important for me to acknowledge my parents. They have been a tremendous influence on the choices I have made that have led me to become a registered dietitian. I appreciate them for tirelessly offering nutritious food to us during childhood, even when it was not the popular thing to do. Finally, I would like to thank my patients, who teach me so much about life.

Foreword

As a practicing internist, over 70 percent of my time is spent treating weight-related diseases. My days are filled with patients whose blood pressure keeps going up just as their waistlines continue to expand, and diabetics whose hard-to-break eating habits necessitate frequent medication adjustments to keep their glucose levels controlled. I keep diagnosing more and more sleep apnea (a condition where people stop breathing at night for short periods due to their abdominal girth pressing on their lungs), and countless people suffering from disabling knee and hip pain as their joints wear out much faster from carrying the weight of all those extra pounds.

With more than 70 percent of the population being overweight or obese, is it any wonder that doctors' offices continue to see so much suffering from obesity-related illnesses? We, as a society, have spent an enormous amount of time and effort educating ourselves on the dangers of such scourges as tobacco smoking, HIV, tuberculosis, and other diseases, yet only recently have we turned our attention to something truly epidemic—obesity, and all the ills brought on by it.

While new medications and technologies will play their roles in the treatment of medical complications, nothing will replace the value of education when it comes to preventing obesity and its related illnesses in the first place. It is critical that more people, and ideally everyone, learn the basics of healthy nutrition. Learning the basics will serve you and your family well for life. What's needed more than ever is for real nutrition professionals to bring clarity and expertise to the field so congested with charlatans, magic potion peddlers, and the latest diet or fat-burner gimmicks.

LeeAnn Smith Weintraub, an experienced registered dietitian, has written just such a book. With years of successful practice counseling patients struggling with weight gain, she channels her knowledge and insight into this practical, how-to guide. From theoretical overview to specific recipes, LeeAnn shows how this critical concept can be implemented in everyday life. This important new book serves as a great foundation and illuminates with great clarity the most important nutritional concept when it comes to fighting and preventing obesity: the glycemic index.

Scientifically proven to improve diabetes control and help lose and maintain weight, a low glycemic index nutrition plan is a must to be learned and followed by anyone interested in healthy ways of eating. Yet this book manages to accomplish much more than just inform you about the scientific merit of the low glycemic index approach—it lavishes you with many delicious, satisfying, and downright scrumptious recipes for every mealtime of the day. Successful weight control relies on clear, reliable information. What more can one ask for than being guided through every meal and snack of the day with plentiful, healthful recipe options? So not only does this book give a great overview of the ideas behind healthy nutrition, it enables you to easily follow and enjoy the path to better health and good taste. Enjoy the book, as I have, and try the recipes that intrigue you—you won't go wrong with any of them. *Bon appétit* and be well!

Ilya M. Rachman, MD, PhD
Clinical Instructor, UCLA David Geffen School of Medicine
Medical Director, Trim360, LLC

Introduction

THERE ARE MANY REASONS for using the glycemic index (GI). The glycemic index has been studied for decades and was originally developed as a dietary strategy in the treatment of diabetes. Today, use of the glycemic index has expanded, and it is now used in the treatment of many common health concerns, including obesity and heart disease. Because it teaches a healthy and balanced way of eating, the GI also has a role in disease prevention. All over the world, people with prediabetes symptoms, excess pounds, and imbalanced diets turn to the GI for assistance in changing their eating habits. Others who can benefit from the GI include women with polycystic ovarian syndrome, individuals with hypoglycemia, and athletes who want to improve performance.

The glycemic index ranks carbohydrate foods based on their impact on blood sugar levels after consumption. The higher the GI level of a food, the faster the spike in blood sugar. Choosing low GI foods helps to control both blood sugar and insulin levels. The first step in using the glycemic index is to know the glycemic index level of different foods.

In the first chapter of the *The Everything® Glycemic Index Cookbook, 2nd Edition*, you will learn about carbohydrate metabolism and how the glycemic index works. You will understand the difference between low and high glycemic index foods. Please refer to the Glycemic Index Value Table at the end of Chapter 1 to get started with meal planning and stocking a GI-friendly pantry.

The following chapters contain recipes that have been created by an experienced registered dietitian. They are designed to be tasty while including a wide variety of low-glycemic ingredients. You will discover recipes for breakfast, lunch, and dinner, as well as appetizers, soups, desserts, and more. Vegetarians will find a nice selection of meat-free options. Each recipe is noted with its glycemic index level category. This book is useful for beginners as well as those experienced with the glycemic index.

Although following the glycemic index is a beneficial way of eating, other factors play an important role in health, longevity, and weight control. The total amount of calories consumed should be considered when planning meals. Understanding serving sizes for portion control will help you become a better judge of how much food to put on your plate. You will notice serving sizes are included in the Glycemic Index Value Table. In addition to eating right, regular physical activity is a necessary part of a balanced lifestyle. Exercise helps burn excess calories that may otherwise be stored as body fat. In addition, regular exercise can decrease the risk of many of the health concerns that are mentioned in this book.

Now that you have decided to improve your health, the glycemic index will help you on your journey. This book will answer your questions and prepare you to make changes in the way you eat. The recipes will provide you with a diverse selection of delicious meals to choose from to stay satisfied.

CHAPTER 1

Understanding the Glycemic Index

The glycemic index (GI) is a useful and effective tool for managing weight and controlling blood sugar levels. Here you will learn how to successfully use the glycemic index in daily meal planning. Knowing how to select low GI foods is the first step to using the glycemic index. This cookbook provides delicious and satisfying recipes for all occasions and appetites to keep you on track with your health and wellness goals.

What Is the Glycemic Index?

The glycemic index is a simple and valuable tool that can be used to help choose the right carbohydrate foods to keep blood sugar levels stable. It is based on a numerical index that ranks foods based on their glycemic response in the body. Lower GI foods are more slowly digested and absorbed and, therefore, produce gentler fluctuations in blood sugar and insulin levels. Higher glycemic index foods cause a quicker rise in blood sugar and insulin. Knowing how to choose the right carbohydrate foods, plan balanced meals, and select the right portion sizes are the keys to weight control, disease prevention, and overall good health.

FACT

Eating controlled portion sizes is a basic part of following any healthy eating plan. The glycemic index is a useful and beneficial tool that is best followed when reasonable serving sizes are eaten at meals and as snacks. Take a look at the serving sizes listed in the Glycemic Index Value Table at the end of the chapter.

The glycemic index levels of foods have been determined by tests performed by scientists in clinical settings. This is done by feeding human test subjects a determined portion of the test food and drawing and testing samples of their blood at specific intervals of time. The test subjects' blood sugar response to a carbohydrate food is compared to the blood sugar response to an equal portion of pure glucose. Glucose, which has a GI level of 100, is the reference food for glycemic index testing. For example, if orange juice is being tested and is found to raise the blood sugar level only 50 percent as much as pure glucose, orange juice is given a glycemic index level of 50. Based on its GI level, a food can be assigned to one of three GI categories: low, moderate, and high glycemic index.

▼ GLYCEMIC INDEX CATEGORIES

Low GI: 55 or less
Moderate GI: 56–69
High GI: 70 or more

It is healthy to eat a wide variety of low-glycemic foods while minimizing higher-glycemic foods. The recipes in this book are categorized as either zero, very low, low, or moderate in the "Per Serving" section. This category is determined based on the glycemic index of the foods combined in the recipe.

Who Can Benefit from the Glycemic Index?

A diet that follows the glycemic index can be beneficial for everyone. This is not a restrictive diet that eliminates major food groups or pushes expensive supplements. Using the GI is a simple way to start eating better now. People with diabetes, metabolic syndrome, and those interested in weight management have a lot to gain from implementing the principles of the glycemic index in their lifestyle. However, a GI diet is not just for those with special health needs; it is a healthy and balanced way of eating for anyone who wants to take care of his or her body, feel good, and experience longevity.

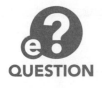

QUESTION

Can I use the glycemic index if I am a vegetarian?
Absolutely! A GI diet is vegetarian-friendly because it allows a variety of plant-based protein foods such as beans, nuts, and tofu. Check out Chapter 9 for delicious vegetarian recipes.

How the Glycemic Index Works

When carbohydrate foods are eaten, the pancreas releases insulin into the bloodstream with the job of carrying sugar into the cells to be used for energy. Intake of high GI foods and general overeating causes elevated circulating insulin levels in the blood. Insulin works to lower blood sugar levels and does this by turning excess sugar into stored fat. When insulin levels are high, the body is not able to burn stored body fat. Even with increased physical activity and exercise, it can be difficult to lose weight when insulin levels are consistently elevated. Elevated blood insulin is also associated with increased appetite, sugar cravings, high blood triglycerides, high blood pressure, heart disease, and diabetes.

Carbohydrate foods include grains, fruits, starchy vegetables, nuts, and legumes. However, not all carbohydrates are nutritionally equal, and they can differ greatly on the glycemic index. Also, common sense cannot always accurately predict the GI level of certain foods. For example, although honey is quite sweet, it actually has a lower GI level than white bread. Research shows that different types of carbohydrates have significantly different effects on blood sugar levels and appetite. Although equal portions of jasmine rice and brown rice have similar amounts of calories, their GI levels are nothing alike. Brown rice, a lower GI food, will have less of an impact on insulin secretion while satisfying hunger.

ALERT

To include desserts and other recipes using sweet ingredients while avoiding high glycemic sugars and sweeteners, alternatives such as agave nectar, Splenda, and fresh fruit are incorporated to satisfy the sweet tooth. Find fun and flavorful dessert recipes in Chapter 16.

Benefits of the Glycemic Index

The primary goal of a diet that follows the glycemic index is to minimize and prevent insulin-related health problems such as diabetes, heart disease, and being overweight by avoiding foods with the largest impact on blood sugar. By keeping blood sugar levels stable, insulin levels remain constant. A low GI diet is often recommended for individuals who are at risk for developing diabetes because of its role in reducing insulin fluctuations.

Eating foods that cause large and fast glycemic response may lead to an initial quick surge in energy, shortly followed by a decrease in blood sugar, which results in lethargy, hunger, mood swings, and fat storage. Replacing high GI foods with low GI foods helps to sustain energy levels throughout the day. A low GI diet that prevents the ups and downs in blood sugar and insulin helps achieve appetite control and mood stability while preventing weight gain.

Limitations of the Glycemic Index

Because it requires participation of human subjects, testing the glycemic index of foods is both expensive and time consuming. Each year thousands of new food products flood the grocery store shelves and, because GI testing is not mandatory, most are not tested. When the GI of a particular food is unknown, the Nutrition Facts food label may be able to provide some clues to help in food selection. Foods that are higher in protein, fat, and dietary fiber while lower in carbohydrates often have a lower GI.

Although GI levels of foods are tested individually, these foods are often eaten with meals in the presence of other foods. The GI level of a meal depends on the GI level of all the foods consumed together. Food preparation technique and food processing also impact the GI level of the meal. The recipes in this cookbook are based on the principle of combining low GI ingredients to create GI-friendly foods and meals.

Carbohydrate Metabolism

In order to better understand why low glycemic index eating is healthful, it is important to be knowledgeable about carbohydrate metabolism. Following are the definitions to some important terms.

Helpful Definitions

Insulin is a natural hormone made by cells in the pancreas, and it is responsible for controlling the level of sugar in the blood. When carbohydrates (sugar) are absorbed in the intestines and enter the bloodstream, blood sugar levels rise. In response to rising blood sugar levels, insulin is secreted, which enables sugar to enter the cells to be used for energy.

Cortisol is a hormone released by the adrenal glands. It works to stabilize blood sugar levels by rising as blood sugar levels fall. High cortisol levels are associated with the storage of body fat around the belly.

Metabolic syndrome is characterized by a group of risk factors for diabetes and heart disease. These risk factors include excessive fat around the abdomen, high blood pressure, abnormal lipid levels (high cholesterol), and insulin resistance.

Insulin resistance is a condition in which the body makes insulin but is unable to use it properly. As a result, the body needs more insulin to help sugar enter the cells. Individuals with insulin resistance have elevated levels of both insulin and sugar in the blood, which increases the risk of developing diabetes and heart disease.

Leptin is a key hormone in energy metabolism. Studies show that low levels of leptin are associated with the accumulation of body fat and diabetes. A low leptin level tells the brain to eat more, and a high leptin level signals satiety or fullness. Individuals with low leptin levels are prone to overeating and gaining weight. Losing weight can help regulate leptin levels.

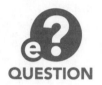

QUESTION

How is metabolic syndrome diagnosed?
Metabolic syndrome is present if three or more of the following risk factors are identified: high serum triglycerides (≥150 mg/dL), reduced HDL "good" cholesterol (men < 40 mg/dL and women < 50 mg/dL), elevated waist circumference, high blood pressure, and high blood sugar.

Glycemic Index versus the Low-Carb Diet

The body requires three types of major nutrients: carbohydrates, fats, and proteins. Carbohydrates are a major source of energy in the diet, one that the brain prefers as fuel.

A low glycemic index diet should not be confused with a low-carbohydrate diet. Low-carb diets restrict many sources of carbohydrate such as breads, potatoes, sweets, fruits, and vegetables in order to put the body in a state of ketosis. In ketosis, the body uses stored fat for energy, and rapid weight loss may occur. However, not only is the potential health risk of such a limited diet a concern, but the long-term sustainability of a high-fat, high-protein diet is highly unlikely. Many people who practice low-carb diets may initially lose weight, but they then gain weight back once returning to old eating habits.

A low GI diet focuses on choosing healthy, low-glycemic foods to promote weight loss and wellness. Fruits, vegetables, beans, nuts, and whole grains, in addition to lean proteins and heart-healthy fats, comprise your meals. Following a low GI diet allows a large variety of readily available nutritious foods; it is more like a way of life than a diet.

ALERT

Because low-carb diets are extremely restrictive, there are potential health concerns that come along with this kind of diet. Restricting fruits and vegetables causes dietary levels of essential nutrients to be inadequate, including vitamins, minerals, antioxidants, phytochemicals, and fiber. Low-carb diets are high in protein and fat, including saturated fat, which may increase the risk of heart disease.

Low GI Carbs Are Good for the Brain

Although the muscles can use either fat or carbohydrate for energy, the brain relies on carbohydrate. Mental performance increases with the consumption of carbohydrate-rich foods. Improved intellectual performance in areas such as short-term memory, mathematics, and reasoning is experienced after eating a carbohydrate meal. This is true for college students, elderly individuals, and even patients with Alzheimer's disease. Studies have shown that memory and intellectual performance improve more with low GI meals compared to meals with high GI carbohydrates.

Food and Appetite

The types of foods you eat dictate how much food you eat. This is because some foods are better than others at suppressing appetite and controlling hunger. Not only quantity, but also quality of food is important to consider for those who want to manage their weight. Foods that contain a lot of calories and fat in a standard serving are referred to as "energy dense." For example, a large chocolate chip cookie can have as much as 500 calories, the same number of calories as six fresh peaches. It is easier to consume excess calories from the cookie than from the six peaches. When eating mostly low energy density foods, your appetite will become suppressed by eating less calories and fat.

How does energy density relate to the glycemic index? The principle of energy density explains why choosing simply a low-fat or low-carb diet for weight control is not the best answer. Often, low-fat foods are supplemented with sugar to make them taste better, and they end up having just as many calories as the alternatives. At the same time, low-carb diets are high in fat, and fat is extremely energy-dense. A diet that utilizes the glycemic index allows for reasonable amounts of carbohydrate, fat, and protein and places more emphasis on the type of fat than the total amount. The glycemic index diet includes many servings of fruits, vegetables, and lower GI carbohydrates—an approach that focuses on the quality of foods.

Glycemic Index and Fiber

Fiber plays an important role in wellness and weight control. There are many benefits to choosing high-fiber foods and eating enough fiber. Studies have shown that the quality of carbohydrates is important in preventing diabetes and controlling appetite. Since high-fiber foods help to improve satiety after meals, eating sufficient amounts of fiber is necessary for weight control. Traditionally, societies that have more plant-based dietary fiber in their cuisine experience less chronic illness.

Do you know how much dietary fiber is recommended daily? The recommended daily amount of dietary fiber is 25 grams for women and 38 grams for men. Americans fall short of these goals with an average usual intake of only 15 grams of fiber per day. Many low GI foods such as whole grains, fresh fruits, and vegetables are excellent sources of fiber.

Principles for Meal Planning

Being well-prepared by keeping low glycemic index foods stocked in the pantry will have you on your way to eating a low GI diet. Plan a weekly menu using the recipes in this book. Go shopping at the market ahead of time to gather the ingredients needed for the recipes.

There are certain ingredients and staple items that you will notice in many of the recipes. It is a good idea to keep these items in stock so you will have a GI-friendly kitchen. Some of these ingredients include agave nectar or syrup, almond flour, whole-wheat flour, olive oil, balsamic vinegar, red wine vinegar, whole-wheat pasta, brown rice, nuts, canned and dry beans, Italian seasoning, garlic, flaxseeds, soy sauce, and Dijon mustard.

LOW GI FOODS

- All nonstarchy vegetables, such as lettuce, broccoli, spinach, onion, and green beans
- Most fruits, including stone fruits, apples, berries, cherries, and citrus fruits
- Nuts, beans, seeds, and legumes
- Plain, unsweetened yogurt and cheese (choose low-fat or nonfat when possible)
- Minimally processed whole grains, such as steel-cut oats, brown rice, whole-wheat and sprouted grain breads, granola and muesli, and whole-wheat pasta

HIGH GI FOODS

- Refined flours and grains
- Processed breakfast cereals
- Sweetened beverages such as soda and juice
- Dried fruits and dates
- Starchy vegetables such as white potatoes, winter squash, and pumpkin
- Refined sugar and sweeteners

Be careful when choosing a food when you are unsure of its glycemic index level. It is best to look foods up before assuming that their GI level is low. For example, grapes have a low GI value, but raisins have a moderate GI value. Take serving size into account as well. For example, a serving size of grapes is 1 cup while it's only ¼ cup for raisins.

Glycemic Index Value Table

GLYCEMIC INDEX VALUES OF COMMON FOODS	
Food and Serving Size	**Glycemic Index Value**
Fruits	
Apple, 1 medium	38
Apple juice, 1 cup	40
Apricots, fresh, 3 medium	57
Apricots, canned, 3 halves	64
Avocado, ¼ cup	<20
Banana, unripe	30
Banana, underripe	51
Banana, overripe	82
Blueberries, 1 cup	40
Cantaloupe, ¼ small	65
Cherries, 10 large	22
Grapes, green, 1 cup	46
Grapefruit, ½ medium	25
Grapefruit juice, 1 cup	48
Kiwi, 1 medium, peeled	52
Mango, 1 small	55
Orange, 1 medium	44
Orange juice, ¾ cup	50
Papaya, ½ medium	58
Peach, 1 medium	42
Peach, canned, ½ cup	30
Pear, 1 medium	38
Pear, canned, ½ cup	44
Pineapple, 2 slices	66
Plum, 1 medium	39
Raspberries, 1 cup	40
Strawberries, 1 cup	40
Watermelon, 1 cup	72
Vegetables	
Acorn squash, ½ cup	75
Bean sprouts, 1 cup	<20
Beets, canned, ½ cup	64
Bell peppers, 1 cup	<20

GLYCEMIC INDEX VALUES OF COMMON FOODS	
Food and Serving Size	**Glycemic Index Value**
Broccoli, 1 cup	<20
Brussels sprouts, 1 cup	<20
Butternut squash, ½ cup	75
Cabbage, 1 cup, raw	<20
Carrots, 1 cup, raw	49
Carrot juice, 1 cup	43
Cauliflower, 1 cup	<20
Celery, 1 cup	<20
Corn, ½ cup	55
Green beans, 1 cup	54
Green peas, 1 cup	48
Parsnips, ½ cup	97
Potatoes, French fried, 4 ounces	75
Potatoes, mashed, ½ cup	74
Potatoes, red-skinned, baked, 4 ounces	93
Potatoes, russet, baked	85
Spaghetti squash, ½ cup	<20
Spinach, 1 cup, raw	<20
Sweet potatoes, boiled, ½ cup	54
Tomato sauce, ½ cup	37
Zucchini, 1 cup	<20
Grains	
Bagel, 1 small, plain	72
Barley, pearled, boiled, ½ cup	25
Banana bread, 1 slice	47
Basmati white rice, boiled, ⅓ cup	58
Brown rice, cooked, ⅓ cup	48
Buckwheat, ⅓ cup	25
Corn tortilla, 1 tortilla	70
Cornmeal, ⅓ cup	68
Couscous, cooked, ½ cup	65
Dark rye bread, 1 slice	76
French baguette, 1 ounce	95
Hamburger bun, 1 item	61
Instant rice, cooked, ½ cup	87
Melba toast, 6 pieces	70

GLYCEMIC INDEX VALUES OF COMMON FOODS	
Food and Serving Size	Glycemic Index Value
Oat-bran bread, 1 slice	44
Oatmeal, cooked, 1 cup	49
Pasta, spaghetti, cooked, 1 cup	41
Pasta, spaghetti, whole wheat, 1 cup	37
Pasta, whole wheat, ½ cup	37
Polenta, boiled	68
Pumpernickel bread, 1 slice	51
Quinoa, boiled	53
Raisin bread, whole grain	44
Rye bread, 1 slice	65
Rye bread, seeded 1 slice	51
Sourdough bread, 1 slice	52
Wheat tortilla, 6", 1 tortilla	30
White bread, 1 slice	70
Whole-wheat bread, 1 slice	69
Dairy and Dairy Alternatives	
Milk, whole, 1 cup	27
Milk, 1%, 1 cup	23
Milk, fat-free, 1 cup	32
Pudding, ½ cup	43
Soy milk, original, 1 cup	44
Soy yogurt, fruit, 2% fat, 1 cup	36
Yogurt, low-fat, berry	28
Yogurt, nonfat, berry	38
Yogurt, nonfat, plain	14
Beans and Nuts	
Baked beans, ½ cup	48
Black beans, boiled, ¾ cup	30
Blackeyed peas, canned, ½ cup	42
Broad beans, ½ cup	79
Cashews, 1 ounce	22
Chickpeas, canned, drained, ½ cup	43
Kidney beans, canned, canned, ½ cup	52
Lentils, boiled, ½ cup	30
Lima beans, ½ cup	32
Mung beans, ½ cup	31

GLYCEMIC INDEX VALUES OF COMMON FOODS	
Food and Serving Size	**Glycemic Index Value**
Peanuts, 1 ounce	15
Pecans, raw, 1 ounce	10
Pinto beans, canned, ½ cup	45
Soybeans, boiled, ½ cup	18
Miscellaneous	
Angel food cake, 1 ounce slice	67
Agave nectar, 1 tablespoon	11
Banana bread, 3-ounce slice	47
Cheese tortellini, cooked	50
Dark chocolate, 1 ounce	41
Honey, 1 tablespoon	58
Maple-flavored syrup, 1 tablespoon	68
Maple syrup, pure, 1 tablespoon	54
Sushi, salmon	48

CHAPTER 2

Breakfast and Brunch

Sunday Morning French Toast

The fiber from the whole-wheat bread and the protein from the eggs make for a complete and satisfying weekend brunch.

INGREDIENTS | SERVES 1

1 tablespoon salted butter
2 eggs
1 tablespoon vanilla extract
1 tablespoon cinnamon
2 slices whole-wheat bread

Low-Cholesterol French Toast

To make this recipe more heart-healthy, decrease the fat and cholesterol by forgetting the egg yolks. Try using ½ cup egg substitute instead of 2 whole eggs. You can find egg substitute near the eggs in the dairy section in the grocery store.

1. Heat a large griddle and brush with butter.

2. Crack eggs into a shallow bowl and beat well with vanilla extract and cinnamon.

3. Cut bread in half diagonally. Dip triangles of whole-wheat bread in the egg mixture, turning once to coat well.

4. Place the bread slices in the pan and cook for 2 minutes on each side, until crisp and golden brown.

PER SERVING: Calories: 438 | GI: Moderate | Carbohydrates: 32g | Protein: 20g | Fat: 23g

Tomato and Feta Frittata

This frittata can be made for a quick and easy breakfast or a relaxed weekend brunch.

INGREDIENTS | SERVES 1

2 egg whites
1 egg with yolk
2 tablespoons crumbled feta cheese
½ cup tomatoes, chopped
Salt and pepper, to taste

Healthy Egg Dish

Quiches taste great, but they are loaded with fat, cholesterol, and calories. Plus, the crust often has a high glycemic value. Frittatas are a GI-friendly and lighter option for a delicious and easy egg dish.

1. Separate 2 egg whites from the yolks and place in a medium bowl. Add 1 whole egg to the bowl with egg whites.

2. Whisk eggs, feta, and tomatoes together.

3. Cook the egg mixture over medium heat in a small skillet coated with cooking spray for 4 minutes or until eggs are firm. Do not stir.

4. Flip and cook the other side for 2 more minutes. Season with salt and pepper to taste.

PER SERVING: Calories: 126 | GI: Very low | Carbohydrates: 6g | Protein: 15g | Fat: 11g

Chicken Breakfast Burrito

This hot and filling breakfast is perfect for a high-protein meal on the go.

INGREDIENTS | SERVES 1

1 tablespoon olive oil

½ cup green bell pepper, chopped

¼ cup onion, chopped

4 ounces chicken breast, diced

1 whole-wheat tortilla

¼ cup salsa

1 tablespoon sour cream

Egg-cellent

For extra protein without all the fat, try adding a scrambled egg white to the chicken burrito. High-protein breakfasts are a healthy start to the day and can help keep you satisfied until the next mealtime.

1. Place a sauté pan on medium-high heat and add olive oil. Combine diced green pepper and onion and sauté in pan for approximately 5 minutes.

2. Add diced chicken to pan and cook until done, about 7 minutes.

3. Top whole-wheat tortilla with chicken and vegetable mixture.

4. Add salsa and sour cream, and then fold tortilla.

PER SERVING: Calories: 467 | GI: Moderate | Carbohydrates: 37g | Protein: 33g | Fat: 21g

Blueberry Oat-Bran Muffins

Here is a healthy spin on the classic blueberry muffin.
Oat bran and flaxseeds boost the fiber in this tasty breakfast bread.

INGREDIENTS | SERVES 8

2 cups oat bran

½ cup soy flour

2 teaspoons baking powder

¼ teaspoon baking soda

½ cup almond flour

½ tablespoon ground nutmeg

1 tablespoon orange zest

¼ cup fructose

¼ teaspoon salt

4 tablespoons cinnamon

2 tablespoons flaxseeds

1 tablespoon unsweetened cocoa powder

½ cup orange juice

2 tablespoons vanilla extract

2 tablespoons vegetable oil

½ cup plain low-fat yogurt

1 cup blueberries

1. Preheat oven to 350°F.

2. Combine dry ingredients and stir to mix well.

3. In a separate bowl, combine wet ingredients, except blueberries, and mix well.

4. Combine wet and dry ingredients, stirring until all ingredients are moist. Fold in blueberries.

5. Spoon into a greased muffin pan or use muffin cups. Spoon equal amounts into each muffin cup. For 12 muffins, bake 20–25 minutes, or until muffin tops are golden brown. For 6 large muffins, increase the cooking time to 40 minutes.

PER SERVING: Calories: 258 | GI: Moderate | Carbohydrates: 40g | Protein: 10g | Fat: 11g

Orange Cranberry Oat-Bran Muffins

Try trading out the blueberries in this recipe for tart fresh or frozen cranberries. Adding an additional teaspoon of orange zest will balance out the flavors nicely. You can use mini muffin pans and a shorter cook time for fun, bite-sized muffins.

Cottage Cheese Pancakes

This batter can be whipped up in a snap for tasty high-protein pancakes or waffles.

INGREDIENTS | SERVES 4

½ cup whole-wheat flour
¼ teaspoon salt
¼ cup olive oil
1 cup low-fat milk
½ teaspoon vanilla extract
6 large eggs
1 cup low-fat cottage cheese
Nonstick cooking spray, as needed

1. Blend all ingredients except cooking spray in a blender until smooth.

2. Spray a pan with nonstick cooking spray and place over medium heat. Pour ¼-cup portions of batter onto hot pan to form pancakes. As the pan heats up, adjust the temperature to prevent the pancakes from becoming too dark.

3. Cook pancakes 2–3 minutes per side until golden brown. Make the pancakes in small batches and, when done, cover to keep warm.

PER SERVING: Calories: 354 | GI: Low | Carbohydrates: 16g | Protein: 21g | Fat: 23g

Blueberry Pancakes

Try adding a few handfuls of blueberries to your pancake batter. Blueberries are an excellent source of antioxidant phytonutrients, called anthocyanidins, that are responsible for the blue-red pigment seen in blueberries. Anthocyanidins help to protect the body from harm from free radicals.

Irish Oatmeal and Poached Fruit

This will keep the kids going for hours! It has the perfect combination of slow-release starch and get 'em going fruit. The nuts will stave off hunger, too!

INGREDIENTS | SERVES 4

1 fresh peach, chopped

½ cup raisins

1 tart apple, cored and chopped

½ cup water

3 tablespoons honey

½ teaspoon salt

2 cups Irish or Scottish oatmeal

1½ cups nonfat milk

1½ cups low-fat yogurt

1 cup toasted walnuts

1. In a saucepan, mix the peach, raisins, and apple with water, honey, and salt. Bring to a boil and remove from heat.

2. Mix the oatmeal and milk with the low-fat yogurt. Cook according to package directions.

3. Mix in the fruit and cook for another 2–3 minutes. Serve hot, sprinkled with walnuts.

> **TIP:** Substitute 1 tablespoon honey for the 3 tablespoons honey and use ½ cup toasted walnuts instead of 1 cup.

PER SERVING: Calories: 600 | GI: Moderate | Carbohydrates: 61g | Protein: 32g | Fat: 36g

Instant Oatmeal

Avoid instant oatmeal for breakfast, for cookies, and for making snacks. The oats in instant oatmeal are cut very thinly, and particle size is important to a low GI. The larger the particles, the lower the food is on the GI.

Sausage and Spicy Eggs

This is a very pretty dish that is not only a delicious breakfast but is also good for lunch or a late supper. Be careful not to overly salt the dish—most sausage has quite a lot of salt in it, so taste first.

INGREDIENTS | SERVES 4

1 pound Italian sweet sausage

¼ cup water

1 tablespoon olive oil

2 sweet red peppers, roasted and chopped

1 jalapeño pepper, seeded and minced

8 eggs

¾ cup 2% milk

2 tablespoons fresh parsley for garnish

1. Cut the sausage in ¼" coins. Place in a heavy frying pan with the water and olive oil. Bring to a boil, then turn down the heat to simmer.

2. When the sausages are brown, remove them to a paper towel. Add the sweet red peppers and jalapeño pepper to the pan and sauté over medium heat for 5 minutes.

3. While the peppers sauté, beat the eggs and milk together vigorously. Add to the pan and gently fold over until puffed and moist.

4. Mix in the reserved sausage, garnish with parsley, and serve hot.

TIP: *Substitute nonfat milk for 2% milk and vegetarian sausage for Italian sweet sausage.*

PER SERVING: Calories: 383 | GI: Low | Carbohydrates: 8g | Protein: 35g | Fat: 23g

Banana Chocolate Pecan Pancakes

This is a rich and luxurious breakfast treat, yet it's low on the GI scale.

INGREDIENTS | SERVES 4

2 1-ounce squares semisweet baker's chocolate

2 tablespoons water

1 cup pecans

1 cup whole-wheat flour

2 teaspoons baking powder

3 eggs, well beaten

¾ cup 2% milk

6 tablespoons honey, or to taste

1 teaspoon pure vanilla extract

½ teaspoon salt

Nonstick spray, as needed

2 bananas, peeled and sliced ¼" thick

Wow, What a Great Brunch Dish!

A morning meal with chocolate and bananas sounds like a decadent treat. Using whole-wheat flour, nuts, and semisweet chocolate instead of milk chocolate helps to keep these pancakes low on the glycemic index without compromising taste.

1. Melt chocolate with water and set aside to cool slightly. Lightly toast the pecans and grind in a food processor, or chop by hand.

2. In a large bowl, mix pecans, flour, and baking powder. Slowly beat in the eggs, milk, honey, vanilla, salt, and then chocolate.

3. Spray a griddle or frying pan with nonstick spray. Heat to medium-high. Drop the pancake batter, about 2 tablespoons per pancake, on the hot griddle. Cover with banana slices. Turn when bubbles form at the top of the cakes.

4. Serve hot with butter, marmalade, or chocolate syrup.

TIP: *Substitute nonfat milk for 2% milk.*

PER SERVING (PLAIN) | Calories: 200 | GI: Low | Carbohydrates: 24g | Protein: 10g | Fat: 7g

Spinach and Gorgonzola Egg-White Omelet

This is diet and comfort food. The two don't seem to go together, but try this!
The quick and easy spinach filling is a frozen spinach soufflé.

INGREDIENTS | SERVES 2

Nonstick butter-flavored cooking spray, as needed

1 frozen spinach soufflé, defrosted

8 egg whites, well beaten

⅛ teaspoon ground nutmeg

1 teaspoon lemon zest, finely grated

½ cup Gorgonzola cheese, crumbled

Salt and pepper, to taste

The Versatile Omelet

The fantastic thing about an omelet is that you can stuff it with all kinds of ingredients. Various veggies, fruits, and cheeses and combinations thereof make exciting omelets. Try mixing some Cheddar cheese sauce and broccoli or some Brie and raspberries for your next omelet and enjoy the flavors!

1. Prepare a nonstick pan with butter-flavored cooking spray. Make sure the spinach soufflé is thoroughly defrosted.

2. Place the pan over medium-high heat. Pour in the beaten egg whites and sprinkle with nutmeg, lemon zest, and cheese. Spoon 1 cup of the spinach soufflé down the middle of the omelet. Reserve the rest for another use.

3. When the omelet starts to set, fold the outsides over the center. Cook until it reaches your desired level of firmness.

PER SERVING: Calories: 463 | GI: Low | Carbohydrates: 16g | Protein: 37g | Fat: 28g

The Vanilla Smoothie Breakfast

This basic smoothie will become a favorite in your house!
Simple and delicious, the wheat bran will fill you up while the yogurt provides calcium.

INGREDIENTS | SERVES 1

1 cup plain low-fat yogurt
1 package sugar substitute
1 teaspoon pure vanilla extract
2 ice cubes
1 tablespoon wheat bran

Place all ingredients in the blender and blend until the ice cubes are pulverized.

PER SERVING: Calories: 262 | GI: Low | Carbohydrates: 11g | Protein: 4g | Fat: 4g

Smoothie with Chocolate and Coffee

At last, a smoothie for grownups! Try this one the next time you are entertaining friends.
Dutch process cocoa is a less acidic unsweetened cocoa.
It is less bitter than natural unsweetened cocoa and blends easily with liquids.

INGREDIENTS | SERVES 2

2 tablespoons instant espresso, dissolved in 2 tablespoons hot water
2 tablespoons Dutch process cocoa, dissolved in ½ cup cold water
1 package sugar substitute, or to taste
½ cup oat bran
1½ cups plain low-fat yogurt
1 tablespoon anisette liqueur, optional
6 ice cubes

When the coffee and cocoa are dissolved, blend all ingredients in the blender and serve.

PER SERVING: Calories: 196 | GI: Low | Carbohydrates: 28g | Protein: 12g | Fat: 6g

Peach and Raspberry Smoothie

The mixture of raspberries and peaches is the basis of classic peach Melba—a wonderful dessert.
This smoothie is rich and always sure to please.

INGREDIENTS | SERVES 2

2 fresh peaches, peeled, pitted, and quartered

1 cup fresh raspberries

1½ cups plain low-fat yogurt

2 packages sugar substitute

1 teaspoon pure vanilla extract

6 ice cubes

2 raw, pasteurized eggs

Place all ingredients in the blender and purée until well blended.

PER SERVING: Calories: 315 | GI: Low | Carbohydrates: 34g | Protein: 88g | Fat: 9g

Quick Breakfast

An easy breakfast for on the go, smoothies are a tasty and nutrient-rich morning pick-me-up. They also make a healthy and satisfying lunch for active and busy lifestyles. For extra protein, you may add a scoop of plain protein powder to the recipe.

Banana-Kiwi Smoothie

Kiwi fruit are delicious, inexpensive, and a bit exotic.
They happen to be loaded with vitamins as well!

INGREDIENTS | SERVES 2

1 banana, peeled, cut in 2" segments

4 kiwi fruit, peeled, cut into halves

Juice of 1 lime

1½ cups orange juice

2 tablespoons oat bran or Kashi

4 ice cubes

Optional—4 drops hot sauce

Place the banana, kiwi, lime juice, and orange juice in the blender and purée. Add the rest and blend until smooth. Serve chilled.

PER SERVING: Calories: 237 | GI: Low | Carbohydrates: 65g | Protein: 10g | Fat: 1g

Smoked Fish and Eggs with Grilled Tomatoes

*This recipe is somewhere between a frittata and an omelet and incorporates
the wonderful flavor of smoked fish into a healthy breakfast.*

INGREDIENTS | SERVES 4

Nonstick butter-flavored spray

4 scallions, chopped

8 eggs

½ cup 2% milk

½ pound smoked salmon or herring, chopped

4 ounces cream cheese, softened

Grilled or Broiled Red Tomatoes (see following recipe)

1. Spray a large frying pan with nonstick spray and add scallions. Sauté the scallions over medium heat until soft, about 3 minutes.

2. Beat the eggs and milk together and stir them into the pan with the scallions. Set the heat on low.

3. Sprinkle the top with salmon or herring and dot with cream cheese. When just set, cut in wedges and serve with grilled red tomatoes.

TIP: *Substitute nonfat milk for 2% milk and low-fat cream cheese instead of regular cream cheese.*

PER SERVING: Calories: 326 | GI: Moderate | Carbohydrates: 3g | Protein: 26g | Fat: 23g

Tomatoes for Breakfast

It seems that all over the British Isles, Spain, and the Mediterranean, you get grilled or broiled tomatoes with meals, from breakfast to dinner. They are perfectly delicious and very nutritious. Americans should have them more often!

Grilled or Broiled Red Tomatoes

This is an excellent side dish to accompany eggs. The tomatoes pick up the flavors of any herbs used with them, and you can add butter, cheese, and spices to flavor the tomatoes in a variety of ways.

INGREDIENTS | SERVES 1

1 large ripe red tomato

1 teaspoon olive oil or butter

1 teaspoon of your favorite herbs (rosemary, parsley, thyme, or basil)

Salt and pepper, to taste

Not Just for Breakfast

Grilled tomatoes also taste great added to salads, soups, or served up with juicy grilled meats and fish. Using ruby red, orange, yellow, and green heirloom tomatoes is a yummy way to add flavor and color to your plate.

1. Cut the tomato in half, from top to bottom. Use a melon baller to remove seeds. Sprinkle with oil, herbs, salt, and pepper.

2. Nest the tomatoes individually in aluminum foil with the top open. Place open-end up on the grill, over indirect heat. Close lid and roast for 15 minutes at 375°F.

PER SERVING: Calories: 67 | GI: Low | Carbohydrates: 6g | Protein: 1g | Fat: 5g

Baked Grapefruit with Honey and Chambord

This is a super-simple starter that never fails to impress brunch guests! The Chambord and honey bring out the sweetness in the warm grapefruit.

INGREDIENTS | SERVES 2

1 large juicy grapefruit

2 teaspoons honey

2 teaspoons Chambord (raspberry liqueur)

1. Preheat broiler to 400°F.

2. Cut the grapefruit in half. Loosen the sections with a grapefruit spoon or short paring knife.

3. Spread the honey over the grapefruit halves. Sprinkle with Chambord. Broil for 10 minutes, but be careful not to burn.

PER SERVING: Calories: 79 | GI: Low | Carbohydrates: 19g | Protein: 1g | Fat: 0g

Herbed Omelet with Vegetables

This omelet is a simple way to add an extra serving of vegetables to your day.

INGREDIENTS | SERVES 2

Cooking spray, as needed

2 cups white mushrooms, sliced

3 tablespoons low-fat milk

2 tablespoons sour cream

Salt and pepper to taste

2 tablespoons green onions, chopped

1 tablespoon chives, chopped

¼ teaspoon dried tarragon

4 egg whites

2 eggs

Low-Fat Alternative

Fresh herbs and mushrooms give this omelet tons of earthy flavor. In the summer use fresh herbs from your own garden. To cut back on saturated fat, try using 6 egg whites and passing on the yolks.

1. Heat a large skillet over medium-high heat and coat with cooking spray. Add mushrooms until soft and liquid evaporates.

2. In a bowl, mix together 1 tablespoon milk, sour cream, salt, and pepper. Whisk well and set aside.

3. In a separate bowl, mix remaining 2 tablespoons milk, green onion, chives, tarragon, egg whites, and eggs in a bowl; stir well.

4. Pour egg mixture into a greased pan over medium-high heat and spread evenly over pan. Once center is cooked, cover egg with mushrooms. Loosen omelet with spatula and fold over.

5. Place omelet on a plate to serve and top with sour cream mixture.

PER SERVING: Calories: 164 | GI: Very low | Carbohydrates: 5g | Protein: 17g | Fat: 9g

Green Chilies and Egg Soufflé

*Excluding the egg yolks from this soufflé helps to reduce saturated fat
for a lighter and healthier breakfast.*

INGREDIENTS | SERVES 2

1 cup egg whites
Salt and pepper to taste
4 tablespoons unsalted butter
½ cup red bell pepper, chopped
3 tablespoons diced green chilies
¼ cup Monterey jack cheese, shredded
½ cup low-fat cottage cheese

Heat It Up!

For a spicier soufflé, add diced jalapeño pepper or Thai chili. Just remember to remove and discard the inner membranes and seeds before chopping the pepper up if you want to keep the heat under control. You may substitute red bell peppers with green, yellow, or orange.

1. Preheat the oven to 400°F.

2. Whip the egg whites to soft peaks, adding salt and pepper to taste.

3. In a heavy 9" oven-safe pan, melt butter over high heat.

4. Add bell peppers and chilies, season lightly, and cook until tender.

5. Immediately fold the cheese and cottage cheese into the whites and spread out evenly over the peppers and chilies. Place in the oven and bake for about 8 minutes until golden on top.

PER SERVING: Calories: 367 | GI: Very low | Carbohydrates: 6g | Protein: 24g | Fat: 28g

Yogurt and Fruit Parfait

This fast and easy breakfast is packed full of calcium, fiber, and antioxidants.

INGREDIENTS | SERVES 1

1 cup nonfat yogurt
¼ cup blueberries
¼ cup strawberries, sliced
4 tablespoons almonds, sliced

Greek Yogurt

Try using Greek yogurt, preferably nonfat or low-fat, for a thicker, richer, and slightly tart parfait. Greek yogurt tastes great with sweet berries. For a simple snack, try adding a teaspoon of honey to plain Greek yogurt. What a treat!

1. Add ½ cup yogurt to tall glass.

2. Layer half the berries and 2 tablespoons of almond slices on top of the yogurt.

3. Place the remaining yogurt on top of the berry and almond layer.

4. Add the remaining berries and 2 tablespoons almonds to the top of the second yogurt layer.

PER SERVING: Calories: 303 | GI: Moderate | Carbohydrates: 32g | Protein: 19g | Fat: 12g

CHAPTER 3

Appetizers

Baked Coconut Shrimp

Agave nectar is used to sweeten the shrimp, keeping this appetizer low on the glycemic index. This lower GI substitute for sugar or honey is derived from the blue agave plant, which thrives in volcanic soils in southern Mexico.

INGREDIENTS | SERVES 8

Cooking spray, as needed

⅓ cup almond flour

½ teaspoon ground red pepper

Salt to taste

Juice of ½ lime

1 tablespoon agave nectar

⅓ cup egg whites

¾ cup coconut

1½ pounds extra-large shrimp, shelled and cleaned with tails remaining

How to Pair Coconut

Coconut is a fun ingredient to work with because it is a delicious island treat. Coconut has the power to sweep the mind away to thoughts of a warm, sandy beach. This ingredient must be paired with the right ingredients to work well in a dish. Some flavors that coconut goes well with include lime, chocolate, pineapple, banana, orange, and shellfish.

1. Preheat oven to 425°F and lightly spray a baking sheet with cooking spray.

2. In a small bowl, combine almond flour, pepper, and salt.

3. In a separate bowl, mix lime juice and agave nectar and stir. Continuously stirring, add egg whites to lime-agave mixture.

4. Place coconut in a thin layer on a flat dish. Dip each shrimp first into the almond flour mixture, then in the egg white mixture, and then roll in coconut.

5. Place on baking sheet. Bake 10–15 minutes or until coconut appears lightly toasted.

PER SERVING: Calories: 173 | GI: Very low | Carbohydrates: 4g | Protein: 20g | Fat: 9g

Fresh Baja Guacamole

*A traditional guacamole is a crowd-pleasing appetizer
or a tasty addition to a simple sandwich or wrap.*

INGREDIENTS | SERVES 4

2 ripe avocados

½ red onion, minced (about ½ cup)

2 tablespoons cilantro leaves, finely chopped

Juice of 1 lime

Salt and freshly grated black pepper, to taste

1 serrano chili, minced

½ tomato, chopped

Working with Hot Chilies

Put on rubber gloves when handling hot chili peppers. They can sting, burn, and irritate the skin. Avoid touching your eyes during or after working with chilies. Be sure to wash your hands with soap and warm water right after.

1. Cut avocados in half. Remove the seed. Scoop avocado away from the peel and place in a mixing bowl.

2. Using a fork to mash avocado. Add the chopped onion, cilantro, lime juice, salt, and pepper. Mix ingredients together.

3. Cut open chili pepper and scrape out stems, seeds, and veins with the tip of a knife. Add to the guacamole to your desired degree of hotness.

4. Add chopped tomatoes just before serving.

PER SERVING: Calories: 133 | GI: Very low | Carbohydrates: 10g | Protein: 2g | Fat: 11g

Baked Chicken Wings

Cayenne pepper is known for its metabolism-boosting properties.
Blended with paprika and garlic, cayenne is sure to kick up the heat in these chicken wings.

INGREDIENTS | SERVES 4

12 chicken wings
3 tablespoons soy sauce
½ tablespoon garlic powder
1 teaspoon paprika
1 teaspoon cayenne pepper
2 teaspoons agave nectar
Salt and pepper to taste
1 tablespoon olive oil

1. Wash the chicken wings and pat dry.

2. Combine remaining ingredients except olive oil in a bowl. Add wings and coat with mixture. Cover and refrigerate for 1–2 hours or overnight.

3. Preheat oven to 425°F. Cover a baking dish with aluminum foil. Drizzle foil with olive oil. Place wings in one layer in baking dish.

4. Bake for 40 minutes or until golden brown. Turn the wings over after 20 minutes to allow even cooking.

PER SERVING: Calories: 211 | GI: Very low | Carbohydrates: 3g | Protein: 18g | Fat: 14g

Pickled String Beans

This cold green bean appetizer is a delicious and healthy start to your meal.
Fresh dill smells beautiful and adds the finishing touch to this dish.

INGREDIENTS | SERVES 4

2 cups green beans, drained
1 cup yellow beans, drained
Juice of 1 lemon
1 teaspoon white wine vinegar
1 teaspoon garlic powder
½ teaspoon dill
2 tablespoons onion, minced

1. Combine all ingredients in a bowl.

2. Serve cold.

PER SERVING: Calories: 28 | GI: Very low | Carbohydrates: 6g | Protein: 2g | Fat: 0g

Yellow Green Beans

Green beans are not always green. They can also be yellow and even purple. Green beans of all colors are rich in vitamins A and C. Despite the different appearance, yellow green beans taste the same as their green counterparts.

Stuffed Zucchini Boats

Zucchini acts as the perfect vessel for this tempting vegetarian appetizer.
A finger food topped with cheese and marinara sauce is a sure crowd-pleaser.

INGREDIENTS | SERVES 2

2 large zucchini squashes

1 teaspoon olive oil

Salt and pepper, to taste

4 ounces ground turkey

¼ cup marinara sauce

2 ounces part-skim ricotta cheese

1 tablespoon Parmesan cheese, shredded

Low-Fat Option

To reduce the total calories and fat in the zucchini boats, choose low-fat or fat-free ricotta cheese. The recipe calls for ground turkey since it is leaner than ground beef. Vegetarians or those looking for a meat-free meal can substitute the ground turkey with ground soy "meat."

1. Set oven rack at upper-middle position and turn broiler to high.

2. Slice each zucchini in half lengthwise. Using a spoon, remove seeds from zucchini halves, creating a hollow center.

3. Rub zucchini with oil and season with salt and pepper to taste. Place on a baking sheet with open side facing up. Broil 8 minutes or until zucchini are fork tender.

4. Meanwhile, brown ground turkey in a medium pan over medium heat.

5. Heat marinara sauce in a small saucepan.

6. Remove zucchini from oven and transfer to platter.

7. Combine ground turkey and marinara sauce. Spread a thin layer of ricotta cheese across zucchini; top with meat sauce. Sprinkle with Parmesan cheese.

PER SERVING: Calories: 272 | GI: Low | Carbohydrates: 27g | Protein: 20g | Fat: 11g

Caponata Baked with Brie

Caponata is a very basic Italian vegetable appetizer, most frequently associated with Sicily. It can be served on bread, crackers, or in a sandwich, and it is wonderful for entertaining.

INGREDIENTS | SERVES 8

1 green pepper, cored and chopped

1 zucchini, chopped

1 small eggplant, chopped

1 sweet red onion, chopped

2 cloves garlic, chopped

½ cup olive oil

1 tablespoon sweet basil, dried

1 teaspoon oregano, dried

Salt and pepper to taste

2 tablespoons capers

10 green olives, seeded, chopped

2 tablespoons red wine vinegar

1 sheet frozen puff pastry, thawed

1 6" round of Brie

1. Sauté the vegetables and garlic in the olive oil over medium heat for 10 minutes. Add the herbs, salt and pepper, capers, olives, and stir in red wine vinegar. Cook for another 5 minutes.

2. Preheat the oven to 350°F. Roll out the pastry. Spread Brie on the pastry and spoon vegetables over all.

3. Bake for 25 to 35 minutes, or until pastry is brown. Cut into manageable, appetizer-sized wedges and serve warm or at room temperature.

PER SERVING: Calories: 232 | GI: Moderate | Carbohydrates: 9g | Protein: 5g | Fat: 21g

Lollipop Lamb Chops

This is an expensive appetizer, but it's worth every penny for a special occasion. Citrus zest in recipes adds pungent flavor. The aromas of orange and lemon zest infuse everything from meats to veggies and dressings.

INGREDIENTS | MAKES 14 LAMB CHOPS

4 cloves garlic

4 tablespoons parsley, minced

3 tablespoons rosemary

Grated zest of ½ lemon

3 tablespoons Dijon mustard

2 tablespoons olive oil

Salt and pepper, to taste

14 baby rib lamb chops, trimmed with long bones left on

1. Blend everything but the chops in a mini food processor or blender.

2. Pour into a large dish and add lamb chops, turning to coat both sides.

3. Broil or grill lamb chops for 3 minutes per side.

PER SERVING: Calories: 268 | GI: Very low | Carbohydrates: 0g | Protein: 34g | Fat: 13g

Crowd Pleaser

Baby lamb chops are the star of the show at parties and special occasions. Your guests will love these delicious finger foods. They are fun to eat like chicken wings but make less of a mess.

Ceviche (Fresh Seafood in Citrus)

This is a classic South and Central American appetizer.
The citrus actually "cooks" the seafood, and everything else is a flavor addition.

INGREDIENTS | SERVES 4

½ pound raw tiny bay scallops

½ pound fresh raw shrimp, peeled and deveined

2 scallions, minced

1 green chili, seeded and minced

Juice of 1 fresh lime

2 tablespoons orange juice

1 tablespoon chili sauce

2 tablespoons parsley or cilantro

Salt and pepper to taste

2 tablespoons olive oil

1. Rinse scallops and pat dry in a paper towel.

2. Mix all ingredients except the olive oil in a nonreactive bowl. Cover and refrigerate for 8 hours or overnight.

3. Just before serving, sprinkle with olive oil. Serve in large cocktail glasses.

PER SERVING: Calories: 159 | GI: Very low | Carbohydrates: 4g | Protein: 18g | Fat: 11g

More about Ceviche

Ceviche is made by using the acid from citrus juice instead of heat to cook fresh seafood. It has been enjoyed in South America for centuries. Ceviche is made differently all over the world, but it typically always contains fish and shellfish. Other common ingredients include thinly sliced onion, hot pepper, orange juice, lemon, garlic, corn, lettuce, and sweet potato.

Stuffed Mushrooms (Crabmeat or Shrimp)

These can be made in advance and frozen. This is very good party fare,
but be sure you make enough—they go quickly!

INGREDIENTS | MAKES 12 INDIVIDUAL
STUFFED MUSHROOMS

¼ pound cooked shrimp or crabmeat
(canned or fresh)

1 cup soft white bread crumbs

½ cup light mayonnaise

Juice of ½ lemon

1 teaspoon fresh dill weed, or 1
teaspoon dried

Salt and pepper to taste

12 mushrooms, 1"–1½" across, stems
removed

1. Mix together everything but the mushrooms.

2. At this point, you can stuff the mushrooms and refrigerate or freeze, or you can continue the recipe.

3. Preheat oven to 400°F. Place stuffed mushrooms on a baking sheet and bake for 15–20 minutes. Serve hot.

PER SERVING: Calories: 103 | GI: Low | Carbohydrates: 5g |
Protein: 3g | Fat: 8g

Buying Mushrooms

Buy only the whitest, crispest mushrooms. If you buy them from a grower, you'll see that they stay white and unblemished for at least three weeks. Old mushrooms are tan to brown with black/brown flecks.

Stuffed Mushrooms (Spicy Beef)

These disappear rapidly at a party—people love them! As in Stuffed Mushrooms (Crabmeat or Shrimp) (see previous recipe), you can make them in advance and either refrigerate or freeze.

INGREDIENTS | MAKES 12 INDIVIDUAL STUFFED MUSHROOMS

2 tablespoons olive oil

¼ pound ground sirloin (very lean)

2 shallots, minced

1 clove garlic, minced

Salt and pepper to taste

1 teaspoon red hot pepper sauce, or to taste

1 teaspoon fresh gingerroot, minced

1 egg

1 teaspoon Worcestershire or other steak sauce

12 mushrooms, 1"–1½" across, stems removed

Nonstick spray, as needed

6 teaspoons fine white bread crumbs

1. Preheat the oven to 400°F. Heat the oil and brown the sirloin, shallots, and garlic. Stir in the seasonings, egg, and Worcestershire sauce. Set aside while you clean and stem the mushrooms.

2. Set mushrooms on a baking sheet that you have prepared with nonstick spray. Stuff mushrooms. Sprinkle with bread crumbs.

3. Bake for 30 minutes, until tops are brown and mushrooms are sizzling.

PER SERVING: Calories: 54 | GI: Low | Carbohydrates: 2g | Protein: 3g | Fat: 4g

Stuffed Mushrooms (Bacon and Herbs)

This is a delicious appetizer at brunch!
You could also serve these on the side with eggs.

INGREDIENTS | MAKES 16 INDIVIDUAL STUFFED MUSHROOMS

16 mushrooms, 1"–1½" across, stems reserved and chopped

Nonstick spray, as needed

2 strips high-quality bacon, cut in small pieces

½ red onion, minced

2 slices whole-wheat bread, toasted and crumbled

Pinch nutmeg

2 teaspoons fresh parsley, minced

2 teaspoons fresh sage, minced

1 egg

1. Preheat the oven to 350°F. Clean mushrooms and place on a baking sheet that you have prepared with a nonstick spray.

2. Sauté bacon, onion, and mushroom stems until the bacon is crisp. Stir in bread crumbs, nutmeg, parsley, and sage. Let cool slightly and mix in the egg.

3. Spoon mixture into mushrooms. Bake for 20 minutes or until lightly browned and very hot.

TIP: *Substitute Canadian bacon or vegetarian bacon for regular bacon.*

PER SERVING: Calories: 23 | GI: Low | Carbohydrates: 3g | Protein: 1g | Fat: 1g

Baked Stuffed Clams

Try to use fresh clams rather than canned in this dish. Once you do, you'll never go back to canned! Cherrystone clams are hard-shell quahogs and are generally 2½" in diameter.

INGREDIENTS | SERVES 4, 2 HALF CLAMS PER PERSON

4 fresh cherrystone clams, well-scrubbed and opened, meat removed

1 tablespoon lemon juice

2 slices whole-grain wheat bread, toasted and crumbled

1 egg

1 tablespoon mayonnaise

½ teaspoon dried dill

2 tablespoons butter, melted

Salt and pepper to taste

2 tablespoons Parmesan cheese

1. Preheat the oven to 350°F. Place the clam shells on a baking sheet.

2. Place the clam meat and the rest of the ingredients in the food processor or blender and pulse until mixed but not puréed.

3. Spoon the stuffing into the clam shells and bake for about 20 minutes. Serve immediately.

> **TIP:** *Substitute 2 tablespoons olive oil or heart-healthy margarine for butter and low-fat mayonnaise for regular mayonnaise.*

PER SERVING: Calories: 195 | GI: Low | Carbohydrates: 11g | Protein: 13g | Fat: 11g

Follow Your Nose and Your Ears!

When buying any kind of seafood, ask to smell it first. A fresh, salty aroma is fine; anything else is suspect—don't buy it! When selecting clams, make sure that they are tightly closed and make a sharp click when you tap them together.

Baked Oysters

*The easiest way to make this is to buy shucked oysters and bake them
in commercially available scallop shells or ramekins.*

INGREDIENTS | SERVES 6

Nonstick spray, as needed

1½ pints shucked oysters, drained

Juice of ½ lemon

1 10-ounce box frozen creamed spinach, drained

Light grating of nutmeg

4 teaspoons Parmesan cheese

1. Spray the shells or ramekins with nonstick spray.

2. Divide the oysters among the shells. Sprinkle with lemon juice. Spoon the creamed spinach over the oysters and grate a bit of nutmeg over the top. Sprinkle with Parmesan cheese.

3. Bake for about 20 minutes, until the oysters are very hot and the cheese topping is lightly browned.

PER SERVING: Calories: 159 | GI: Moderate | Carbohydrates: 10g | Protein: 9g | Fat: 7g

Stuffed Celery

*This unique take on stuffed celery is wonderful, replacing peanut butter
or cream cheese with luxurious, buttery Brie.*

**INGREDIENTS | MAKES 12 PIECES
STUFFED CELERY**

Wide ends of 6 celery stalks, cut into halves

5 ounces Brie cheese, softened

2 tablespoons capers

3 tablespoons chopped walnuts, toasted

1. Lay the celery pieces on a cool serving plate. Remove the skin from the Brie then mash with a fork. Mix in the capers.

2. Stuff each piece of celery and garnish with toasted walnuts.

PER SERVING: Calories: 66 | GI: Low | Carbohydrates: 1g | Protein: 3g | Fat: 6g

Clams Casino

This is great with tiny littleneck clams, which are sweet and tasty. Some are saltier than others, so between the combination of the clams and bacon, do not add any salt at all.

INGREDIENTS | SERVES 4

16 littleneck clams, opened, juices retained

4 tablespoons butter

1 small onion, finely minced

Juice of ½ fresh lemon

2 teaspoons fresh parsley, chopped

½ teaspoon dried oregano

½ cup roasted sweet red pepper, finely chopped

3 tablespoons fine white bread crumbs

Freshly ground black pepper to taste

3 slices bacon, cut into 1" pieces

1. Preheat oven to 400°F. Place the open clams on a baking pan.

2. In a saucepan over medium heat, add the butter, onion, lemon juice, herbs, and red pepper. Mix well when butter melts and sauté for about 4 minutes. Mix in bread crumbs and sprinkle with pepper. Moisten with reserved clam juice.

3. Divide the bread crumb mixture among the clams.

4. Put a piece of bacon on top of each stuffed clam. Bake for 12 minutes, or until the bacon is crisp and the clams are bubbling.

TIP: *To reduce the amount of saturated fat and salt, Canadian bacon or vegetarian bacon can be used instead of regular bacon.*

PER SERVING: Calories: 238 | GI: Low | Carbohydrates: 11g | Protein: 11g | Fat: 17g

Deviled Eggs with Capers

If deviled eggs aren't spicy, they aren't devilish enough! This recipe can be adapted if you want less heat. Deviled eggs are easy to make and transport—great for a picnic or brunch!

INGREDIENTS | MAKES 12 HALF EGGS

6 hard-boiled eggs, shelled and cut in half
½ cup low-fat mayonnaise
1 teaspoon Tabasco
1 teaspoon celery salt
1 teaspoon onion powder
1 teaspoon garlic powder
1 chili pepper, finely minced, or to taste
2 tablespoons capers, extra small
Garnish of paprika or chopped chives

1. Scoop out egg yolks and place in food processor along with mayonnaise, Tabasco, celery salt, onion powder, garlic powder, chili pepper, and capers. Blend until smooth and spoon into the hollows in the eggs.

2. Add the garnish of paprika or chives and chill, covered, with aluminum foil tented above the egg yolk mixture.

PER SERVING: Calories: 69 | GI: Low | Carbohydrates: 0g | Protein: 3g | Fat: 6g

Brine-Packed Capers

Capers are actually berries that have been pickled. You can get them packed in salt, but they are better when packed in brine. You can get larger ones or very, very small ones—the tiny ones are tastier.

Maryland Crab Cakes

You can use imitation crabmeat in this recipe, but it's better to use fresh.

INGREDIENTS | SERVES 4

1 pound lump crabmeat

¼ cup mayonnaise

¼ cup soft white bread crumbs

Juice of ½ lemon

1 egg

Salt and pepper to taste

2 tablespoons fresh parsley, chopped

½ cup canola oil, for frying

Tartar sauce, to taste

1. Mix together all ingredients but the oil and tartar sauce and form into cakes.

2. Heat the oil in the frying pan to 275°F. Fry the cakes until well browned on both sides. Serve with tartar sauce.

> **TIP:** *In this recipe you can substitute low-fat mayonnaise for regular mayonnaise and use cooking spray instead of canola oil.*

PER SERVING: Calories: 494 | GI: Low | Carbohydrates: 4g | Protein: 25g | Fat: 43g

Crab Cake Tips

The trick to making the best crab cakes is not skimping on the crab meat. Using fresh lump crabmeat will show through in the final result. Lemon juice and pepper serve to perk up the overall seafood flavor. Tartar sauce is a traditional condiment for crab cakes, but for a change try serving them with the Cajun Rémoulade (see Chapter 14).

Marinated Baby Artichoke Hearts

Here's where frozen artichoke hearts work perfectly! They save you the time and energy of cutting out the choke and removing the leaves of fresh artichokes, and they taste delicious when marinated.

INGREDIENTS | SERVES 4

2 9-ounce or 10-ounce boxes frozen artichoke hearts

½ cup white wine vinegar

¼ cup olive oil

1 teaspoon Dijon-style mustard

½ teaspoon ground coriander seeds

Salt and freshly ground black pepper to taste

1. Thaw and cook the artichokes according to package directions. Drain and set aside.

2. Whisk the rest of the ingredients together in a bowl large enough to hold the artichokes. Add the warm artichokes and cover with dressing. Cover and marinate for 2–4 hours. Serve as antipasto.

PER SERVING: Calories: 142 | GI: Very low | Carbohydrates: 4g | Protein: 1g | Fat: 15g

Mini Codfish Cakes

These are a wonderful appetizer, served with tartar sauce or Aioli (see Chapter 14).

INGREDIENTS | MAKES 12 SMALL CODFISH CAKES

Juice of ½ lemon

½ cup water

1 pound boneless, skinless fillet of cod

1 egg

3 slices good white bread

1 teaspoon dill weed

½ cup mayonnaise

Salt and pepper to taste

½ cup fine white bread crumbs

½" light oil, such as canola, in frying pan

1. Bring lemon juice and water to boil, then add fish and boil until it flakes, about 8 minutes. Drain and cool.

2. Put the fish, egg, bread, dill, mayonnaise, salt, and pepper in the food processor or blender and pulse until coarsely mixed. Turn out onto waxed paper.

3. Form into small cakes and sprinkle with bread crumbs.

4. Heat oil to 350°F and fry cakes until well browned. Serve hot or warm.

TIP: *Substitute low-fat mayonnaise for regular mayonnaise.*

PER SERVING: Calories: 303 | GI: Low | Carbohydrates: 6g | Protein: 10g | Fat: 27g

Baked Stuffed Artichokes

These are worth a bit of effort. You can make them in advance, then finish cooking just before serving.

INGREDIENTS | SERVES 4

2 large artichokes

2 tablespoons olive oil

2 cloves garlic, chopped

½ sweet onion, chopped

1 cup whole-grain cracker crumbs, made in the food processor or blender

1 tablespoon lemon peel, minced

8 medium shrimp, peeled and deveined

4 tablespoons fresh parsley

½ teaspoon freshly ground black pepper, or to taste

4 quarts plus ½ cup water

Juice and rind of ½ lemon

½ teaspoon ground coriander seed

1 tablespoon Parmesan cheese

1. Remove any tough or brown outside leaves from the artichokes. Using a sharp knife, cut off artichoke tops, about ½" down. Slam the artichokes against a countertop to loosen leaves. Cut in half, from top to stem, and set aside.

2. Heat the olive oil in a large frying pan over medium heat. Add the garlic and onion and sauté for 5 minutes, stirring. Add the cracker crumbs, lemon peel, shrimp, parsley, and pepper. Cook until shrimp turns pink. Pulse in the food processor or blender.

3. Boil the artichokes in 4 quarts water with lemon and coriander for 18 minutes. Place the artichokes in a baking dish with ½ cup water on the bottom. Pile with shrimp filling. Drizzle with a bit of the cooking water, sprinkle with Parmesan cheese, and bake for 25 minutes.

PER SERVING: Calories: 403 | GI: Moderate | Carbohydrates: 54g | Protein: 15g | Fat: 16g

CHAPTER 4

Entrée Salads for Lunch and Dinner

Texas Caviar

*This super-simple bean salad is enough to feed a small crowd at a potluck or picnic.
Serve with grilled meat hot off the barbecue and a fresh green salad.*

INGREDIENTS | SERVES 8

1 pound black-eyed peas
Water, as needed
1½ cups Italian salad dressing
1 cup white corn
2 cups red bell peppers, diced
1½ cups onion, diced
1 cup green onions, finely chopped
½ cup jalapeño peppers, finely chopped
1 tablespoon garlic, finely chopped
Salt and Tabasco to taste

Timesaving Tip

You may substitute 2 12-ounce cans of black-eyed peas for 1 pound of dried peas and use your favorite bottled salad dressing to speed up the preparation time. The final result will turn out just as well.

1. Soak peas in enough water to cover for 6 hours or overnight. Drain well.

2. Transfer peas to saucepan. Add water to cover. Place over high heat and bring to boil. Let boil until tender, about 40 minutes; do not overcook.

3. Drain peas well. Transfer peas to a large bowl. Stir in dressing and let cool.

4. Add all remaining ingredients and mix well.

PER SERVING: Calories: 224 | GI: Low | Carbohydrates: 25g | Protein: 3g | Fat: 13g

Avocado and Shrimp Salad

Creamy avocado and refreshing citrus bring out the sweetness of shrimp.
This is a salad you will want to have again and again.

INGREDIENTS | SERVES 4

24 raw shrimp

2 tablespoons olive oil

4 whole green onions, sliced

2 garlic cloves, finely minced

2 tablespoons dry white wine

Salt and pepper to taste

1 red grapefruit

8 ounces butter lettuce, washed and torn into bite-sized piece

1 ripe avocado, sliced

1. Peel and devein the shrimp.

2. In a pan set over medium-high heat, add the olive oil. Add shrimp and half of the green onions to hot pan. Cook, stirring frequently until shrimp are cooked half through. Add minced garlic and white wine to the pan; cook for an additional minute, then add salt and pepper.

3. Cut grapefruit in half and set one half to the side. Add in juice of half grapefruit to the pan; cook for 2 to 3 minutes. Cut the peel off the remaining grapefruit half and slice fruit into bite-sized pieces.

4. Place lettuce, avocado slices, and remaining green onions on salad plates for serving. Transfer cooked shrimp to plates.

5. Drizzle sauce from pan over top and garnish with remaining grapefruit slices.

PER SERVING: Calories: 200 | GI: Low | Carbohydrates: 13g | Protein: 10g | Fat: 13g

Greek Salad

Olives are a rich source of oleic acid, a heart-healthy monounsaturated fat. While various types of olives are commonly used in Mediterranean dishes, Greek salads often feature Kalamata olives.

INGREDIENTS | SERVES 4

4 cups romaine lettuce, chopped into small pieces

1 large tomato, seeds removed and chopped

1 small cucumber, sliced

1 green bell pepper, cut into rings

½ cup feta cheese

¼ cup red wine vinegar

Juice of 1 lemon

1 tablespoon Italian seasoning

Salt and pepper to taste

¼ cup extra-virgin olive oil

2 teaspoons capers

16 Kalamata olives

1. Place lettuce, tomato, cucumber, bell pepper, and feta in a large bowl.

2. To make dressing, whisk vinegar, lemon juice, Italian seasoning, salt, and pepper in a small bowl; mix in olive oil.

3. Coat vegetables with dressing.

4. Place salad on plates. Top salad plates with capers and olives.

PER SERVING: Calories: 228 | GI: Low | Carbohydrates: 20g | Protein: 5g | Fat: 7g

Feta Is "Betta"

Feta cheese has been made by Greek shepherds for centuries. Originally it was made from goat's or sheep's milk; today feta cheese is made from pasteurized cow's milk. In Greece, feta cheese is served in restaurants and homes as a garnish on various types of fresh salads.

Cucumber Salad with Yogurt and Dill

This cool and refreshing salad pairs well with a spicy grilled meat for a relaxing summer barbecue.

INGREDIENTS | SERVES 2

2 large cucumbers
1 cup plain low-fat yogurt
1 tablespoon white wine vinegar
2 tablespoons fresh dill, finely chopped
Salt and pepper, to taste

Making a Cucumber Raita

This recipe may be modified to make raita, an Indian cuisine condiment. Chop the cucumber into ¼" cubes. Substitute the dill with 2 tablespoons chopped mint leaves; add a minced garlic clove and cayenne pepper to taste.

1. Wash and peel cucumbers; chop into ¼"-thick slices.

2. Combine cucumber with yogurt, vinegar, dill, salt, and pepper.

3. Serve chilled.

PER SERVING: Calories: 109 | GI: Low | Carbohydrates: 14g | Protein: 8g | Fat: 2g

Chicken Salad

This salad is the perfect lunch made with extra chicken from last night's dinner.

INGREDIENTS | SERVES 4

1 head romaine lettuce

¼ cup red wine vinegar

2 cloves garlic, minced

2 tablespoons Dijon mustard

1 teaspoon dried rosemary

Salt and pepper to taste

¼ cup olive oil

¼ cup carrot, diced

1 medium red bell pepper, cut lengthwise and minced

¼ cup radish, sliced

2 cups shredded cooked chicken breast

1. Wash romaine lettuce, remove core, and chop leaves into 1" pieces.

2. Combine vinegar, garlic, mustard, rosemary, salt, and pepper in small bowl. Whisk olive oil into vinegar mixture.

3. Place romaine, carrot, bell pepper, radish, and chicken in a large bowl. Pour dressing over salad and toss to coat.

PER SERVING: Calories: 281 | GI: Low | Carbohydrates: 9g | Protein: 24g | Fat: 17g

Not Your Typical Chicken Salad

Using herbs and vegetables brightens up the typical deli-style chicken salad. The purpose of carrots, radishes, bell pepper, and herbs is to spruce up the color on your plate, add crunch, and increase the amount of essential vitamins and fiber.

Blood Orange Salad with Shrimp and Baby Spinach

For an elegant supper or luncheon salad, this is a crowd-pleaser.
The deep red flesh of the blood oranges contrasted with the saturated green of
spinach and the bright pink shrimp makes for a dramatic presentation!

INGREDIENTS | SERVES 4

2 bags baby spinach (try to find prewashed)

2 blood oranges

1¼ pounds shrimp, peeled, deveined, cooked, and chilled

Juice of ½ lemon

¼ cup extra-virgin olive oil

¼ teaspoon dry mustard

Salt and pepper, to taste

¼ cup stemmed, loosely packed parsley or cilantro

1. Just before serving, place the spinach on individual serving plates.

2. Peel the oranges. Slice them crossways, about ¼"-thick, picking out any seeds. Arrange on top of the spinach. Arrange the shrimp around the oranges.

3. Place the rest of the ingredients in the blender and purée until the dressing is bright green. Pour over the salads. Serve chilled.

PER SERVING: Calories: 314 | GI: Low | Carbohydrates: 14g | Protein: 32g | Fat: 16g

Fresh Spinach—Not Lettuce

Substitute fresh baby spinach for less nutritious iceberg lettuce. White or pale green lettuce can be used as accents but have less nutritional substance than such greens as spinach, escarole, chicory, and watercress.

Crabmeat Salad with Rice and Asian Spices

This seafood salad makes a wonderful main course for lunch or supper. Mild and delicious, napa or Chinese cabbage keeps well in the refrigerator and adds an excellent crunch in salads.

INGREDIENTS | SERVES 4

2 cups napa cabbage, shredded

2 cups cooked rice, brown or basmati

1 pound lump crabmeat, fresh (any kind)

1 cup low-fat mayonnaise

2 tablespoons Champagne vinegar

2 tablespoons lemon juice

1 tablespoon sesame seed oil

¼ teaspoon Asian five-spice powder

Salt and pepper, to taste

In a large serving bowl, toss the cabbage, rice, and crabmeat. Mix together the rest of the ingredients for dressing and coat the contents of the bowl. Serve chilled.

PER SERVING: Calories: 471 | GI: Moderate | Carbohydrates: 35g | Protein: 27g | Fat: 25g

Exploring Vinegar

Champagne vinegar is made from the same Champagne used for drinking. It is aged in oak barrels, and because it is made from light, sparkling wine, it has a bright, crisp taste that is delicious in vinaigrettes.

Turkey Club Salad with Bacon, Lettuce, and Tomato

This is a satisfying lunch salad, delicious and easy to make.
You can also put it on a bun and serve it as a sandwich.

INGREDIENTS | SERVES 4

1 pound deli turkey breast

4 strips bacon

1 box cherry tomatoes, halved

1 ripe avocado, peeled and diced

½ cup low-fat mayonnaise

½ cup French Dressing (see Chapter 6)

2 cups lettuce, shredded

Thickly dice turkey breast. Fry bacon until crisp and crumble into large serving bowl. Mix all ingredients except the lettuce in the bowl. Serve over lettuce.

TIP: *For this recipe you can either omit the bacon or substitute it with vegetarian bacon or Canadian bacon.*

PER SERVING: Calories: 518 | GI: Low | Carbohydrates: 14g | Protein: 40g | Fat: 34g

Salad Dressings

Did you ever study the labels of commercial salad dressings? There are chemicals and preservatives in these dressings that you may not want to ingest. Save a nice clean bottle from olives. Make your own dressing and know that everything in it is healthy!

Portobello Mushroom Salad with Gorgonzola, Peppers, and Bacon

The hot Gorgonzola cheese sets this salad apart as an impressive main course or lunch.

INGREDIENTS | SERVES 4

2 large portobello mushrooms
½ cup French Dressing (see Chapter 6)
4 strips bacon
4 ounces Gorgonzola cheese, crumbled
½ cup low-fat mayonnaise
2 cups romaine lettuce, chopped
½ cup sweet red roasted peppers, chopped

Mushroom Choices

There are many varieties of mushrooms now available. Brown mushrooms have a robust flavor. White button mushrooms are delicious in sauces, and the big ones work well when stuffed or grilled. Get wild mushrooms from a reputable mycologist. Never guess if a wild mushroom that you find in the woods is safe. It may be poisonous!

1. Marinate mushrooms for 1 hour in the French dressing. Fry the bacon until crisp; set on paper towels and crumble.

2. On a hot grill or broiler, grill the mushrooms for 3 minutes per side. Cut them in strips.

3. While the mushrooms are cooking, heat the Gorgonzola cheese and mayonnaise in a small saucepan until the cheese melts.

4. Place the mushrooms on the bed of lettuce. Sprinkle with bacon. Drizzle with the cheese mixture and garnish with red roasted peppers.

> **TIP:** *You can make this recipe lower in fat by substituting your favorite low-fat cheese for the Gorgonzola and by using vegetarian "bacon" or Canadian bacon.*

PER SERVING: Calories: 365 | GI: Very low | Carbohydrates: 12g | Protein: 11g | Fat: 31g

Grilled Tuna Salad with Asian Vegetables and Spicy Dressing

The fish is hot, the vegetables are spicy, and the greens are chilled!
This is an exotic salad that is deceptively easy to make.

INGREDIENTS | SERVES 4

3 tablespoons sesame oil

½ cup olive oil

2 cloves garlic, minced

1 teaspoon fresh ginger, minced

2 teaspoons sherry vinegar

1 tablespoon soy sauce

2–3 cups napa cabbage, shredded

1 red onion, cut in wedges

2 Japanese eggplants, cut lengthwise

4 ¼-pound tuna steaks

A Quick Meal

Tuna is a large fish in the mackerel family that has a unique circulatory system that allows them to retain a higher body temperature than the cool waters they inhabit. This provides tuna with an extra burst of energy that allows them to reach short-distance swimming speeds of over 40 miles per hour!

1. In a bowl, whisk together the sesame oil, olive oil, garlic, ginger, sherry vinegar, and soy sauce. Set aside.

2. Place the cabbage on serving plates. Paint the onion, eggplants, and tuna with the dressing, being careful not to contaminate the dressing with a spoon that touched the fish.

3. Grill the vegetables and tuna for 3–4 minutes per side. Arrange the vegetables and fish over the cabbage. Drizzle with the reserved dressing from the second bowl.

PER SERVING: Calories: 388 | GI: Low | Carbohydrates: 13g | Protein: 3g | Fat: 39g

Marinated Chicken and Brown Rice Salad with Water Chestnuts

Some salads, though not fattening, still are very filling. This is one!

INGREDIENTS | SERVES 4

½ cup red wine vinegar

1 cup low-fat mayonnaise

1 teaspoon Dijon-style mustard

½ teaspoon celery salt

4 skinless and boneless chicken breasts, about 4 ounces each

2 cups brown rice, cooked

4 scallions, chopped

1 carrot, julienned

1 8-ounce can water chestnuts, drained and sliced

Salt and pepper, to taste

1 bag mixed greens, washed and ready to use

1. Mix the red wine vinegar, mayonnaise, mustard, and celery salt together in a bowl. Spread 4 teaspoons of the mixture on the chicken breasts, being careful not to contaminate the dressing with a spoon that touched the chicken.

2. Combine the rest of the dressing with the cooked rice. Mix in the scallions, carrot, water chestnuts, salt, and pepper. Set aside.

3. Grill the chicken for about 4–5 minutes per side over high heat. Let rest for 5 minutes and slice.

4. Place the mixed greens on serving plates, mound the rice, and decorate with the warm chicken.

PER SERVING: Calories: 333 | GI: Low | Carbohydrates: 33g | Protein: 5g | Fat: 21g

What Is a Water Chestnut?

A water chestnut is not a nut at all; it's a tuber. Commonly referred to as a Chinese water chestnut, they get their name from a resemblance to a chestnut's shape and color. They grow in freshwater ponds, lakes, and slow-running streams in Japan, China, Thailand, and Australia. Water chestnuts are useful for adding a crunchy texture to recipes such as stir-fries, salads, and stuffing.

Wheat Berry Salad

Highly nutritious and full of vitamins and fiber, this salad is ideal for breakfast or as a side. Wheat berries are whole kernels of wheat that have a hearty, nut-like flavor.

INGREDIENTS | SERVES 6

4 cups water

1 teaspoon kosher salt

1 cup wheat berries

1 cup French Dressing (see Chapter 6)

2 cups jicama (Mexican turnip), peeled and diced

1 green apple, peeled, cored, and diced

½ pound small red grapes, seedless

2 cups mixed baby greens (prewashed)

Freshly ground black pepper to taste

The Homely Legume

Jicama, also known as a Mexican turnip, is a lumpy root vegetable with a unique and versatile taste. The jicama's peel is inedible, but like a potato, it can be fried, baked, boiled, steamed, or mashed. The jicama can also be eaten raw. Try it as a vehicle for guacamole or use its mild flavor and crunchy texture in fruit salad.

1. Bring the water to a boil. Add salt and wheat berries.

2. Cook the wheat berries until crisp/tender, following package directions.

3. Place cooked wheat berries in a large serving bowl. While still warm, toss with the French Dressing. Add jicama, apple, and grapes. Toss and chill. Place mixture on plates over mixed baby greens. Add pepper to taste.

PER SERVING: Calories: 205 | GI: Low | Carbohydrates: 17g | Protein: 1g | Fat: 13g

Fig and Parmesan Curl Salad

This mixture may sound a bit different, and it is!
In addition to being unique, it is also very delicious!

INGREDIENTS | SERVES 2

4 fresh figs, cut into halves, or 4 dried figs, plumped in 1 cup boiling water and soaked for ½ hour

2 cups fresh baby spinach, stems removed

¼ cup olive oil

Juice of ½ lemon

2 tablespoons balsamic vinegar

1 teaspoon honey

1 teaspoon dark brown mustard

Salt and pepper to taste

4 large curls Parmesan cheese

1. When the figs (if dried) are softened, prepare the spinach and arrange on serving dishes.

2. Whisk the olive oil, lemon juice, balsamic vinegar, honey, mustard, salt, and pepper together. Make Parmesan curls with a vegetable peeler and place over figs and spinach; drizzle with dressing.

PER SERVING: Calories: 284 | GI: Low | Carbohydrates: 30g | Protein: 11g | Fat: 16g

A Hidden Gem

Figs are a wonderfully nutritious food. Not only are they high in fiber and minerals, they also add tons of flavor to any recipe. Some cultures even claim that figs have medicinal value and healing potential.

Lentil Salad

This is a salad with a burst of protein from lentils.
Serve as a side or as a main lunch course.

INGREDIENTS | SERVES 4

1 1-pound bag lentils (green, yellow, or red)

Water, as needed

1 medium onion, chopped

½ cup wine vinegar

Salt, to taste

1 diced carrot

2 stalks celery, chopped

2 medium tomatoes, sliced

1 cup French Dressing (see Chapter 6)

1. Cover the lentils with water in a saucepan and add onion and wine vinegar. Bring to a boil, lower heat, and simmer until soft. Sprinkle with salt.

2. Toss with diced carrot and chopped celery and arrange tomatoes around mound of lentils. Sprinkle with French Dressing and serve warm or at room temperature.

PER SERVING: Calories: 287 | GI: Very low | Carbohydrates: 25g | Protein: 7g | Fat: 20g

A Note about Lentils

Like other legumes, lentils are an excellent source of dietary fiber and protein. Due to their small size, lentils cook faster than other beans and legumes. Dried lentils can keep well in the pantry for up to 1 year.

Baby Vegetable Salad

Use the smallest vegetables available for this salad.
Garnish with spicy prosciutto and sweet fennel.

INGREDIENTS | SERVES 4

¼ cup olive oil

2 cloves garlic, minced

12 tiny fresh white onions

1 pound tiny haricots verts

1 bulb fennel, rimmed of any brown and thinly sliced

5 ounces small white button mushrooms

8 baby carrots

¼ cup Champagne vinegar

¼ cup fresh basil, shredded

¼ cup fresh parsley, shredded

Salt and pepper, to taste

½ cup stemmed, loosely packed watercress

1 head Boston lettuce, shredded

½ pound currant or grape tomatoes

½ pound Black Forest ham, chopped

1. Heat the olive oil over medium-low flame and sauté the garlic, onions, haricots verts, fennel, mushrooms, and carrots until the haricots verts and carrots are crisp-tender.

2. Stir in the Champagne vinegar, basil, and parsley. Sprinkle with salt and pepper to taste.

3. When the vegetables are at room temperature, arrange the watercress and lettuce on serving plates and spoon on the veggies. Add tomatoes. Sprinkle with the ham and serve.

PER SERVING: Calories: 346 | GI: Low | Carbohydrates: 18g | Protein: 19g | Fat: 20g

Poached Salmon Salad with Hard-Boiled Eggs

*This is marvelous for summer because you can poach the salmon the night before,
chill it until ready to serve, and have a wonderful cold entrée. Adjust the amount of salmon
to the number of guests invited, adding ¼ to ⅓ pound per person and an extra egg per person.*

INGREDIENTS | SERVES 4

1⅓ pounds salmon fillet, skin and bones removed

½ cup cold water

¼ cup dry white wine

Juice of ½ lemon

1 tablespoon juniper berries, bruised with a mortar and pestle

1 cup low-fat mayonnaise

¼ cup stemmed, loosely packed fresh parsley

2 sprigs fresh dill weed, or 2 teaspoons dried

Zest and juice of ½ lemon

4 drops Tabasco sauce, or to taste

Watercress or lettuce, for arrangement on platter

4 hard-boiled eggs, peeled and sliced

Capers, for garnish

1. Place the salmon in a pan that will hold it without curling the end. Add the water, wine, lemon juice, and juniper berries. Over medium-low heat, poach the fish until it flakes, about 12 minutes, depending on thickness. Do not turn. Drain and cool; refrigerate until just before serving.

2. Put the mayonnaise, parsley, dill, lemon zest and juice, and Tabasco in a blender. Purée until very smooth.

3. Arrange the salmon on a serving platter. Surround with watercress or lettuce and eggs. Dot with capers and serve green mayonnaise on the side.

PER SERVING: Calories: 480 | GI: Low | Carbohydrates: 7g | Protein: 36g | Fat: 33g

Filet Mignon and Red Onion Salad

There are few things that taste better cold than filet mignon!
Use a light salad dressing as both marinade and dressing.

INGREDIENTS | SERVES 4

1¼ pounds well-trimmed whole filet mignon

Salt and pepper, to taste

½ cup French Dressing (see Chapter 6)

1 red onion, thinly sliced

2 tablespoons capers

16 black olives, pitted and sliced

Bed of romaine lettuce, chopped

Know Your Beef

Filet mignon is French for "small and bone-less meat." This cut is the small part of a beef tenderloin and is considered the most delectable cut of beef because of its melt-in-your-mouth texture. Save yourself some money by preparing this at home instead of dining out!

1. Preheat oven to 400°F. Place the filet mignon on a baking pan. Sprinkle it with salt and pepper. Roast for 15 minutes. Rest the meat for 10 minutes before carving.

2. Slice the filet mignon and place in a bowl with the French dressing, onion, capers, and olives. Toss gently to coat.

3. Spread the lettuce on a serving platter. Arrange the filet mignon, onion, olives, and capers over the top. Serve at room temperature or chilled.

PER SERVING: Calories: 501 | GI: Very low | Carbohydrates: 6g | Protein: 41g | Fat: 34g

Fresh Tuna Salad à la Niçoise

The niçoise salad originates from Nice, a French city on the Mediterranean Sea.
This salad is popular in France, like the Cobb salad is enjoyed in the United States.

INGREDIENTS | SERVES 2

¼ pound green beans, trimmed

Water, as needed

2 4-ounce tuna steaks

2 tablespoons olive oil

Salt and pepper, to taste

1 head butter lettuce

1½ tablespoons capers

¼ cup niçoise olives

½ cup cherry tomatoes

2 tablespoons Italian dressing

2 hard-boiled eggs, quartered

Timesaving Tip

If you are tight on time and money, try substituting the tuna steaks with a large can of albacore tuna. Canned albacore usually contains more omega-3 fatty acids than chunk light tuna. The salad will still taste authentic without spending extra cash and time grilling the fish.

1. Cook green beans in a pot of boiling water, uncovered, until crisp-tender, about 4 minutes, then transfer immediately to a bowl of ice water to stop cooking. Drain green beans and pat dry.

2. Brush tuna with olive oil and season with salt and pepper as desired. Grill on lightly oiled rack or grill pan, uncovered, turning over once, until browned on outside and pink in the center, 6–8 minutes total. Slice tuna into ¼"-thick pieces.

3. Wash lettuce and tear into bite-sized pieces; place in large bowl. Add green beans, capers, olives, and tomatoes to bowl; coat with Italian dressing.

4. Divide salad onto two plates. Top with tuna and egg quarters.

PER SERVING: Calories: 430 | GI: Very low | Carbohydrates: 35g | Protein: 8g | Fat: 29g

Arugula and Fennel Salad with Pomegranate

Pomegranates pack a high dose of beneficial health-promoting antioxidants.
They are in peak season October through January and can be substituted with
dried cranberries if unavailable at your local market.

INGREDIENTS | SERVES 4

2 large navel oranges

1 pomegranate

4 cups arugula

1 cup fennel, thinly sliced

4 tablespoons olive oil

Salt and pepper, to taste

Fennel Facts

Fennel, a crunchy and slightly sweet vegetable, is a popular Mediterranean ingredient. Fennel has a white or greenish-white bulb and long stalks with feathery green leaves stemming from the top. Fennel is closely related to cilantro, dill, carrots, and parsley.

1. Cut the tops and bottoms off of the oranges and then cut the remaining peel away from the oranges. Slice each orange into 10–12 small pieces.

2. Remove seeds from the pomegranate.

3. Place arugula, orange pieces, pomegranate seeds, and fennel slices into a large bowl.

4. Coat the salad with olive oil and season with salt and pepper as desired.

PER SERVING: Calories: 224 | GI: Low | Carbohydrates: 24g | Protein: 3g | Fat: 15g

CHAPTER 5

Soups

Vegetable Chili

A steaming hot bowl of this spicy chili will satisfy meat eaters and vegetarians alike.

INGREDIENTS | SERVES 8

2 tablespoons olive oil

1 medium onion, chopped

1 celery stalk, chopped

1 green bell pepper, chopped

1 red bell pepper, chopped

4 cloves garlic, minced

2 tablespoons chipotles in adobo, chopped

1 tablespoon ground cumin

1 tablespoon dried oregano

1 tablespoon chili powder

1½ teaspoons salt

1 28-ounce can diced tomatoes

3 cups water

1½ cups black beans, cooked and drained

3 cups kidney beans, cooked and drained

½ cup sour cream

1. Heat oil in a large pot over medium heat.

2. Add onion, celery, peppers, and garlic, and cook for 10 minutes.

3. Add chipotles, cumin, oregano, chili powder, and salt. Stir ingredients together. Add tomatoes and water. Bring heat down to low, and simmer, uncovered, for 45 minutes.

4. Add beans and simmer for 20 minutes more.

5. Serve with a dollop of sour cream.

PER SERVING: Calories: 230 | GI: Moderate | Carbohydrates: 37g | Protein: 11g | Fat: 5g

Green Pea Soup

This rich and velvety soup will warm you up from the inside out.

INGREDIENTS | SERVES 4

2 tablespoons olive oil

1 medium onion

3 cloves garlic, minced

4 cups chicken stock

3 cups green peas

¾ teaspoon tarragon

¼ tablespoon black pepper

2 slices bacon

4 teaspoons sour cream

1. Heat oil in a pot over medium heat, and add onion and garlic. Cook for 5 minutes or until the onion is soft and translucent.

2. Add chicken stock, peas, and tarragon to pot. Bring to boil, then reduce heat to simmer for 8 minutes.

3. Remove from heat, allow to cool slightly, then purée soup in a food processor or blender. Season the soup with pepper.

4. Place bacon under a broiler and cook until crispy.

5. Serve soup garnished with crumbled bacon and sour cream.

PER SERVING: Calories: 290 | GI: Moderate | Carbohydrates: 28g | Protein: 14g | Fat: 14g

Creamy Cauliflower Soup

Cauliflower, a cruciferous vegetable, contains compounds that may prevent cancer.

INGREDIENTS | SERVES 4

2 tablespoons olive oil
½ cup onion, finely chopped
½ cup celery, chopped
1 cup cauliflower
4 cups chicken stock
1 cup Cheddar cheese, shredded
Salt and pepper, to taste
1 cup low-fat milk

1. Heat oil in a large pot, and sauté onion and celery until translucent. Add cauliflower and chicken stock, and bring to a boil. Reduce heat, cover, and simmer for 25 minutes, stirring occasionally.

2. Purée soup in food processor or blender until smooth.

3. Return soup to pot and bring temperature to medium-low heat. Add cheese, salt, and pepper, continue to cook and stir until cheese is melted and well integrated.

4. Add milk and stir into the soup. Add more chicken stock if the consistency of the soup is too thick.

PER SERVING: Calories: 291 | GI: Low | Carbohydrates: 16g | Protein: 17g | Fat: 18g

Chicken and Rice Soup

This comforting soup stands alone as a healthy and satisfying meal.

INGREDIENTS | SERVES 6

3 boneless, skinless chicken breasts

Salt and pepper, to taste

4 tablespoons olive oil

1 small onion, chopped

2 cloves garlic, minced

3 stalks celery, chopped

2 carrots, peeled and chopped

5½ cups chicken broth

¾ tablespoon thyme

2 cups cabbage, shredded

2 bay leaves

1 cup water

¾ cup long-grain brown rice

Nutrition Note

Chicken and rice soup is a classic American comfort food. Egg noodles have been replaced with brown rice and high-glycemic veggies have been omitted to keep the soup low on the glycemic index and extremely flavorful. This is a guilt-free meal!

1. Wash chicken and pat dry. Season with salt and pepper and chop into 1"-thick pieces.

2. Heat 2 tablespoons oil in pan and sauté chicken pieces for 6–8 minutes, until chicken is well done. Set chicken aside for later.

3. Heat remaining oil in a large pot, and sauté onion and garlic over medium heat until translucent. Add celery and carrot to pot and cook for 5 minutes.

4. Add chicken broth, thyme, cooked chicken, cabbage, bay leaves, water, and rice to the pot. Simmer soup for 30 minutes or until rice is completely cooked. Remove bay leaves before serving.

PER SERVING: Calories: 263 | GI: Low | Carbohydrates: 19g | Protein: 24g | Fat: 10g

Avocado Soup, Chilled with Lime Float

Most cold soups can also be served hot—avocado soup is an exception.
Avocados can be delicious cooked, but this cold soup is too perfect to change.

INGREDIENTS | SERVES 2

2 ripe avocados, peeled

½ cup chicken broth

½ cup buttermilk (nonfat can be used)

Juice of ½ lime

2 shallots, minced

½ teaspoon salt, or to taste

½ cup sour cream

1 teaspoon lime juice

Zest of ½ lime

Tabasco sauce, to taste

1. In the blender, purée the avocados with chicken broth, buttermilk, lime juice, shallots, and salt. Taste for seasoning.

2. Whisk the sour cream, lime juice, lime zest, and Tabasco together. Float on top of the soup.

3. Serve icy cold.

TIP: *Substitute low-fat sour cream for regular sour cream.*

PER SERVING: Calories: 487 | GI: Very low | Carbohydrates: 23g | Protein: 6g | Fat: 45g

Zesty!

While zests are a fabulous way to add a kick of citrus flavor to almost any dish, be careful of lime zest—it gets very bitter when cooked. It is still a wonderful addition to fresh and uncooked dishes.

Cold Basil and Fresh Tomato Soup

This is a wonderful summer soup served cold, or heated for a cold day. It is also good for you!
The red tomatoes are full of vitamin C. (The amount of vitamin C in tomatoes increases as they ripen.)
This soup also freezes beautifully!

INGREDIENTS | SERVES 4

2 pounds red, ripe tomatoes, halved and cored

1 cup beef broth

¼ cup red wine

1 teaspoon garlic powder

20 basil leaves

Salt and pepper, to taste

Chopped chives, for garnish

1. In the blender, purée tomatoes, beef broth, wine, garlic powder, basil, salt, and pepper. Chill overnight. Add garnish at the last minute.

2. If serving the soup hot, garnish with grated Cheddar or Parmesan cheese.

PER SERVING: Calories: 60 | GI: Very low | Carbohydrates: 11g | Protein: 2g | Fat: 0g

Cucumber Soup

Some recipes for cucumber soup call for cooking the cucumber.
This one "cooks" it in the acidity of lemon juice.

INGREDIENTS | SERVES 2

1 slender English cucumber, peeled and chopped

Juice of 1 lemon

1 cup nonfat buttermilk

1 cup low-fat yogurt

2 tablespoons fresh dill weed, snipped

Salt and freshly ground white pepper, to taste

1 teaspoon Tabasco, optional

Garnish of extra snippets of dill or chives

Skin Health

Silica, a chemical known for improving the health and complexion of skin, is found in cucumber juice. Cucumber is used to treat puffy eyes and ease sunburn. Other compounds in cucumbers are said to prevent water retention and dermatitis. Cool cucumbers are soothing and refreshing.

1. Mix all ingredients together except garnish and purée in the blender until smooth. Place in a glass or other nonreactive bowl (to avoid staining a reactive bowl with the acidic citrus).

2. Let rest in the refrigerator for 4 hours or overnight.

3. Taste and add seasonings if necessary before serving in chilled bowls, topped with garnish.

PER SERVING: Calories: 145 | GI: Very low | Carbohydrates: 21g | Protein: 11g | Fat: 3g

Black Bean Soup with Chilies

You can soak your black beans overnight and then cook for 2–3 hours or until tender. Canned beans also work well in this recipe. It's important to adjust the type of chilies to your personal taste. Serrano and Scotch bonnets are among the hottest.

INGREDIENTS | SERVES 4

4 strips bacon

4 cloves garlic, chopped

1 medium sweet onion, chopped

2 hot chilies, seeded and minced

2 cans black beans or 1 pound black beans

8 ounces beef broth

½ cup tomato juice

2 ounces dark rum

Salt and black pepper, to taste

Garnish of fresh lime wedges, sour cream, chopped cilantro, and pepper jack cheese

1. In a large pot, fry the bacon until crisp. Remove bacon to a paper-towel–lined plate and leave the bacon fat in the pot. Crumble bacon. Add garlic, onion, and chilies to the pot. Sauté until softened, about 5 minutes.

2. Stir in the black beans, beef broth, tomato juice, rum, salt, and pepper. Cover and simmer for 1 hour.

3. You may either purée the soup or serve it as is. Garnish with any or all of the suggestions.

PER SERVING: Calories: 206 | GI: Low | Carbohydrates: 27g | Protein: 11g | Fat: 5g

Heart-Healthy Substitution

Beans make for a very nutritious meal. You have a few options to make this recipe more heart-healthy. Instead of bacon, flavor the soup with a ham bone (which you must remove before puréeing or serving) or use vegetarian "bacon."

Broccoli Soup with Cheese

There is a lot to love about broccoli soup. Both nourishing and full of fiber,
it can be enriched with cream or heated up with spicy pepper jack cheese.

INGREDIENTS | SERVES 4

¼ cup olive oil

1 medium sweet onion, chopped

2 cloves garlic, chopped

1 large baking potato, peeled and chopped

1 large bunch broccoli, coarsely chopped

½ cup dry white wine

3 cups chicken broth

Salt and pepper, to taste

Pinch ground nutmeg

4 heaping tablespoons extra sharp Cheddar, grated, for garnish

1. Heat the olive oil in a large soup kettle. Sauté the onion, garlic, and potato over medium heat until softened slightly. Add the broccoli, liquids, and seasonings.

2. Cover the soup and simmer over low heat for 45 minutes.

3. Cool slightly. Purée in the blender. Reheat and place in bowls.

4. Spoon the cheese over the hot soup to serve.

PER SERVING: Calories: 297 | GI: Very low | Carbohydrates: 22g | Protein: 8g | Fat: 19g

Save the Stalks

When you prepare broccoli, save the stems. They can be grated and mixed with carrots in a slaw, cut into coins and served hot, or cooked and puréed as a side. Broccoli marries well with potatoes and carrots and is good served raw with a dipping sauce.

Leek and Potato Soup (Hot or Cold)

There are many versions of this excellent soup, which tastes wonderful when served either hot or chilled. Some recipes have chunky potatoes, and others are smooth— you can prepare this one whichever way you prefer.

INGREDIENTS | SERVES 4

¼ cup olive oil

2 leeks, coarsely chopped

1 large sweet onion, chopped

2 large baking potatoes, peeled and chopped

2 cups chicken broth

1 teaspoon salt, plus more to taste

1 cup 2% milk

1 cup whipping cream

¼ cup chopped chives

Freshly ground pepper, to taste

Garnish of ¼ cup chopped watercress

1. Heat the olive oil in a large soup kettle. Be sure to rinse the sand out of the leeks. Add the leeks and onion and sauté for 5 minutes over medium heat.

2. Add the potatoes, chicken broth, and 1 teaspoon salt. Simmer until the potatoes are tender. Set aside and cool.

3. Put the soup through a ricer or purée in the blender until smooth.

4. Pour the soup back into the pot; add the milk, whipping cream, and chives and reheat. Add salt and pepper to taste. Float the watercress on top for garnish.

TIP: *Replace 2% milk with nonfat milk.*

PER SERVING: Calories: 491 | GI: Moderate | Carbohydrates: 40g | Protein: 8g | Fat: 33g

Onion Soup with Poached Egg Float

This makes a wonderful midnight supper.
Make the soup in advance, and then after heating it, add the eggs.

INGREDIENTS | SERVES 2

2 tablespoons olive oil

½ sweet red onion, chopped

½ sweet white onion, chopped

2 shallots, chopped

2¾ cups rich beef broth

2 tablespoons port wine

1 bay leaf

1 teaspoon Worcestershire sauce

Salt and pepper, to taste

4 eggs

1. Heat the olive oil in a large saucepan. Add the onions and shallots. Sauté for 6 minutes. Add the beef broth, wine, bay leaf, and Worcestershire sauce. Cover and reduce heat to low. Simmer for 30 minutes.

2. Remove bay leaves and add salt and pepper to taste. You can chill the soup until just before serving.

3. Heat the soup. Carefully drop in the eggs and poach for 2 minutes. Serve soup with eggs floating on top.

PER SERVING: Calories: 392 | GI: Very low | Carbohydrates: 23g | Protein: 9g | Fat: 15g

Onions, Shallots, and Chives

When it comes to onions, the more varieties the merrier! When you use several different varieties, you get a depth of flavor that would not be possible if you just use one kind of onion—so mix it up!

Egg Drop Soup with Lemon

This is a lovely spicy version of the Chinese staple, made with a variety of Asian sauces. Asian fish sauce is a liquid made from salted fish that is used in place of salt in many Asian recipes. Hoisin sauce is made from crushed soybeans and garlic, has a sweet and spicy flavor, and is a rich brown color.

INGREDIENTS | SERVES 2

1 tablespoon peanut oil

1 clove garlic, minced

2 cups chicken broth

Juice of ½ lemon

1 tablespoon hoisin sauce

1 teaspoon soy sauce

1 teaspoon Asian fish sauce

½ teaspoon chili oil, or to taste

1" fresh gingerroot, peeled and minced

2 eggs

1. Heat the peanut oil in a large saucepan. Sauté the garlic over medium heat until softened, about 5 minutes.

2. Add chicken broth, lemon juice, hoisin sauce, soy sauce, fish sauce, chili oil, and gingerroot. Stir and cover. Cook over low heat for 20 minutes.

3. Just before serving, whisk the eggs with a fork. Add to the boiling soup and continue to whisk until the eggs form thin strands.

PER SERVING: Calories: 158 | GI: Very low | Carbohydrates: 2g | Protein: 5g | Fat: 13g

Yellow Pepper and Tomato Soup

Yellow peppers and yellow tomatoes are very sweet and make a wonderful soup!

INGREDIENTS | SERVES 4

¼ cup peanut oil

½ cup sweet white onion, chopped

2 cloves garlic, minced

1 sweet yellow bell pepper, finely chopped

1½ cups chicken broth

4 medium-sized yellow tomatoes, cored and puréed

½ teaspoon cumin, ground

½ teaspoon coriander, ground

Juice of ½ lemon

Salt and pepper, to taste

Garnish of fresh basil leaves, torn

1. In a soup kettle, heat the oil over medium flame and sauté the onion, garlic, and yellow pepper. After about 5 minutes add the chicken broth and tomatoes.

2. Stir in the seasonings, lemon juice, salt, and pepper.

3. Cover and simmer. You can purée the soup if you wish or leave some bits of texture in it.

4. Serve hot or cold and sprinkle with basil.

PER SERVING: Calories: 176 | GI: Very low | Carbohydrates: 12g | Protein: 2g | Fat: 14g

Colorful Veggies

Yellow fruits and vegetables are loaded with vitamin A, or retinol, which keeps your skin moist and helps your eyes adjust to changes in light. It is important to eat a variety of different colored fruits and vegetables every day.

Spinach and Sausage Soup with Pink Beans

This is a hearty and delicious soup. If you don't want to work with fresh spinach, get a package of frozen, chopped spinach. You can also substitute escarole or kale. Some sausage is so lean that you will need to add a bit of oil when you cook it.

INGREDIENTS | SERVES 4

8 ounces Italian sweet sausage, cut in bite-sized chunks

2 cups water

¼ cup olive oil

2 white onions, chopped

4 cloves garlic, chopped

2 stalks celery, chopped, leaves included

2 cups beef broth

Bunch fresh spinach, kale, or escarole, or 10-ounce package frozen, chopped spinach

1 teaspoon dried oregano

1 teaspoon red pepper flakes

1 13-ounce can pink or red kidney beans, drained

Salt, to taste

Grated Parmesan cheese, to taste

1. Place the sausage in a soup kettle. Add ¾ cup water and bring to a boil; let water boil off. Add the oil if dry and sauté the onions, garlic, and celery for 10 minutes over medium-low heat.

2. Stir in the rest of the ingredients except the cheese; cover and simmer for 35 minutes. Serve in heated bowls. Garnish with grated Parmesan cheese.

PER SERVING: Calories: 344 | GI: Very low | Carbohydrates: 28g | Protein: 19g | Fat: 20g

Vegetarian Option

This recipe can easily be transformed into a vegetarian-friendly soup. Substitute vegetarian sausage for regular sausage Italian sausage and use vegetable broth instead of beef broth.

Lentil Soup with Winter Vegetables

This is a substantial soup that will get you through a long winter!

INGREDIENTS | SERVES 4

½ pound bag red or yellow lentils

4 cups vegetable broth

2 cups water

2 parsnips, peeled and chopped

2 carrots, peeled and chopped

2 white onions, chopped

4 cloves garlic, chopped

4 small bluenose turnips, peeled and chopped

½ pound deli baked ham, cut in cubes

Put all ingredients in a soup kettle, bring to a boil, cover, and simmer for 1 hour.

PER SERVING: Calories: 188 | GI: Low | Carbohydrates: 19g | Protein: 18g | Fat: 5g

Pumpkin Soup (Slightly Sweet)

If you have a sweet tooth, you can add some more brown sugar to this recipe.

INGREDIENTS | SERVES 4

1 cup Vidalia or other sweet onion, finely chopped

½" fresh gingerroot, peeled and minced

2 cups orange juice

2 cups chicken broth

1 13-ounce can pumpkin (unflavored)

1 teaspoon brown sugar

½ teaspoon ground cinnamon

¼ teaspoon ground nutmeg

¼ teaspoon ground cloves

Optional: ½ cup heavy cream

Stir the ingredients into the soup pot, one by one, whisking after each addition. Cover and simmer for 10 minutes. If you decide to use the cream, add at the last minute.

PER SERVING: Calories: 102 (with heavy cream, add 100 calories) | GI: Low | Carbohydrates: 24g | Protein: 4g | Fat: 0g

Mediterranean Seafood Soup

This quick and easy soup will give you a taste of the Mediterranean.

INGREDIENTS | SERVES 2

2 tablespoons olive oil

½ cup sweet onion, chopped

2 cloves garlic, chopped

½ bulb fennel, chopped

½ cup dry white wine

1 cup clam broth (canned is fine)

2 cups tomatoes, chopped

6 littleneck clams, tightly closed

6 mussels, tightly closed

8 raw shrimp, jumbo, peeled and deveined

1 teaspoon dried basil, or 5 leaves fresh basil, torn

Salt and red pepper flakes, to taste

1. Heat the oil over medium flame and add onion, garlic, and fennel. After 10 minutes, stir in the wine and clam broth and add the tomatoes. Bring to a boil.

2. Drop clams into the boiling liquid. When clams start to open, add the mussels. When mussels start to open, add the shrimp, basil, salt, and pepper flakes. Serve when shrimp turns pink.

PER SERVING: Calories: 450 | GI: Very low | Carbohydrates: 19g | Protein: 48g | Fat: 18g

Littleneck Clams

Littleneck clams are the smallest variety of hard-shell clams and can be found on the northeastern and northwestern coasts of the United States. They have a sweet taste and are delicious steamed and dipped in melted butter, battered and fried, or baked.

Pumpkin Soup (Savory)

Pumpkin soup is fine any time of year. You can always use canned pumpkin, which is very good and easier than peeling and cooking fresh pumpkin. Be sure to buy unsweetened and unflavored pumpkin so that you don't end up with soup tasting like pumpkin pie!

INGREDIENTS | SERVES 4

1 teaspoon butter

1 cup yellow onion, chopped

1½ cups chicken broth

¼ cup dry white wine

1 teaspoon sage leaves, dried, or 4 fresh sage leaves, chopped

½ teaspoon oregano, dried

2 cups canned pumpkin (unflavored)

Salt, to taste

1 teaspoon Tabasco sauce

½ cup heavy cream

Garnish with ⅛ pound smoked ham, chopped

Garnish of chopped fresh chives

1. Melt the butter in a soup kettle and sauté the onion over medium-low heat for 5 minutes. Stir in all but the heavy cream and ham.

2. Simmer the soup, covered, for 10 minutes. Add heavy cream and serve hot with ham and chives sprinkled on top.

> **TIP:** *Substitute olive oil for butter and whole milk for heavy cream.*

PER SERVING: Calories: 166 | GI: Low | Carbohydrates: 9g | Protein: 2g | Fat: 13g

Beef, Barley, and Vegetable Soup

This hearty soup can be made ahead of time and served to a hungry crowd at a wintertime get-together.

INGREDIENTS | SERVES 8

1 tablespoon olive oil

1 pound top round beef, cubed

8 cups beef broth

1 8-ounce can tomato sauce

1½ cups carrots, chopped

1½ cups peas

1½ cups green beans, trimmed

1½ cups barley

4 cloves garlic, minced

1 tablespoon onion powder

Salt and pepper, to taste

1. Heat olive oil in a large pot over medium heat. Add beef cubes to pot and brown.

2. Add broth and tomato sauce and simmer for 1 hour.

3. Add carrots, peas, green beans, barley, garlic, and onion powder to the pot.

4. Simmer for 45 minutes, until barley is cooked. Add salt and pepper as desired.

PER SERVING: Calories: 290 | GI: Moderate | Carbohydrates: 30g | Protein: 28g | Fat: 6g

Barley and Lentil Soup

Lentils are packed with nutrients and are relatively easy to prepare.
Try this soup for a filling cold-weather meal.

INGREDIENTS | SERVES 8

½ cup olive oil

1 cup onion, diced

3 cloves garlic, minced

4 stalks celery, chopped

4 carrots, peeled and thinly sliced

6 cups beef broth

1 28-ounce can tomatoes

¾ cup lentils

¾ cup barley

3 sprigs fresh rosemary

2 tablespoons fresh oregano

Ground black pepper, to taste

About Barley

A versatile grain with a slightly nutty flavor, barley has a pasta-like texture but with loads of fiber. Barley can be used in many different types of recipes as a replacement for white rice and other high GI foods.

1. Heat olive oil in a large pot over low-medium heat. Add onion, garlic, celery, and carrots to hot oil. Stir vegetables to coat with oil and cook until they are soft, about 30 minutes, continuing to stir.

2. Add broth and tomatoes to vegetables.

3. Add lentils, barley, fresh herbs, and black pepper. Stir to mix well.

4. Cover the pot and cook soup on low-medium heat for 45 minutes, making sure that the barley is cooked.

PER SERVING: Calories: 409 | GI: Moderate | Carbohydrates: 33g | Protein: 24g | Fat: 20g

Cashew-Zucchini Soup

Cashews make this soup thick and creamy and provide a serving of heart-healthy fat.

INGREDIENTS | SERVES 4

5 medium zucchini
Nonstick cooking spray, as needed
1 large Vidalia onion, chopped
4 cloves garlic, chopped
½ teaspoon salt
¼ teaspoon ground pepper
3 cups vegetable broth
½ cup raw cashews
½ teaspoon dried tarragon
Additional salt and pepper, to taste

Cashew Nut Butter

To save time you may substitute whole raw cashews with cashew nut butter. You can enjoy using the leftover cashew nut butter as a spread on sandwiches and as a dip for fresh fruit. Remember when snacking on nut butters that they are high in calories, so limit the portion size.

1. Coarsely chop 4 zucchini, leaving 1 zucchini set aside.

2. Spray a large saucepan with nonstick cooking spray. Add onion to the pan and cook for 5 minutes, until soft and translucent. Add garlic and cook for 1 minute. Stir in chopped zucchini, ½ teaspoon salt, and ¼ teaspoon ground pepper and cook over medium heat, covered, occasionally stirring, for 5 minutes.

3. Add the broth and simmer for 15 minutes.

4. Add cashews and tarragon. Purée soup in blender in 1 to 2 batches. Fill blender up to halfway to avoid burns from the hot liquid.

5. Return soup to the pot; season with additional salt and pepper as desired.

PER SERVING: Calories: 117 | GI: Low | Carbohydrates: 23g | Protein: 6g | Fat: 8g

Healthy Snacks and Dips

Spicy Cilantro Dip

Keep edamame, or soybeans, in the freezer so this tasty dip can be easily whipped up for unexpected guests.

INGREDIENTS | SERVES 6

2 cups edamame

1 cup low-fat sour cream

3 tablespoons red wine vinegar

¼ cup lime juice

1 tablespoon olive oil

1 jalapeño, diced

1 bunch fresh cilantro leaves, chopped

1 red bell pepper, chopped

2 shallots, diced

¼ teaspoon salt

¼ teaspoon black pepper

1. Shell edamame.

2. Combine sour cream, vinegar, lime juice, and olive oil and purée in a blender or food processor until smooth.

3. Add edamame, jalapeño, cilantro, red bell pepper, shallots, salt, and pepper to the sour cream mixture and blend to a chunky texture.

4. Serve dip chilled.

PER SERVING: Calories: 135 | GI: Very low | Carbohydrates: 9g | Protein: 6g | Fat: 9g

Timesaving Tip

Edamame, or soybeans, are rich in iron, fiber, omega-3 fatty acids, and many other nutrients. Buy edamame that has already been removed from the shell to save time during preparation. Shelled edamame can often be found in the freezer section at the supermarket.

Mushroom Spread

The mushrooms in this vegetarian spread provide a meaty flavor.
Mushrooms are known for their umami, or savory, taste.

INGREDIENTS | SERVES 4

2 tablespoons olive oil
1 small shallot, chopped
3 cups white mushrooms, sliced
¼ cup cream cheese
¼ cup dry sherry
2 cups flat-leaf parsley
Salt and pepper, to taste
1 zucchini, sliced
1 yellow squash, sliced
1 carrot, sliced

1. Heat oil in a pan and cook shallot until soft. Add mushrooms and cook until water is removed.

2. Blend mushrooms and shallot with cream cheese and sherry in a food processor until smooth. Add parsley, salt, and pepper to food processor and blend well.

3. Serve with grilled or raw vegetable slices.

PER SERVING: Calories: 158 | GI: Low | Carbohydrates: 11g | Protein: 5g | Fat: 10g

Dry Sherry Substitute

Sherry is a fortified wine that comes from southern Spain. It is considered an aperitif and is often served chilled. If you do not have dry sherry on hand, orange juice, pineapple juice, and nonalcoholic vanilla extract are considered good substitutes in correct proportions.

Bean Salsa

This zesty and colorful salsa may be served alone or with a spicy southwestern dish.

INGREDIENTS | SERVES 8

4 cups tomatoes, chopped
2 cups black beans, cooked
1 cup onion, diced
1 jalapeño, seeded and diced
½ cup fresh cilantro, chopped
Juice of 2 limes
Salt and pepper, to taste

1. Mix tomatoes, beans, onion, jalapeño, cilantro, and lime juice in a medium bowl.

2. Add salt and pepper as desired.

PER SERVING: Calories: 84 | GI: Low | Carbohydrates: 17g | Protein: 5g | Fat: 0g

Banana Nut Bread

*This is a low GI take on traditional homemade banana bread
without compromising taste or quality.*

INGREDIENTS | SERVES 8

1½ cups whole-wheat flour

1 teaspoon baking powder

1 teaspoon baking soda

1 tablespoon ground cinnamon

1 tablespoon unsalted butter, melted

4 bananas, mashed

1 large egg

1 teaspoon vanilla extract

⅓ cup Splenda No Calorie Sweetener, granulated

1 cup walnuts, chopped

1. Combine flour, baking powder, baking soda, and cinnamon in a large mixing bowl.

2. Mix butter, mashed bananas, egg, vanilla, and Splenda in a medium mixing bowl.

3. Add banana mixture to flour mixture, stirring to moisten dry ingredients. Mix in walnuts.

4. Pour batter into a greased loaf pan. Bake at 350°F for 50–55 minutes.

PER SERVING: Calories: 241 | GI: Moderate | Carbohydrates: 32g | Protein: 6g | Fat: 12g

Heart-Healthy Walnuts

Walnuts are flavorful and add a nice crunch to cakes and cookies. Because they are an excellent source of omega-3 fatty acids—more so than most other nuts—they are super heart-healthy and good for you.

Fruit Skewers with Dip

A forkless version of the fruit salad, this appetizer can be made with a variety of seasonal fruits.

INGREDIENTS | SERVES 4

4 kiwi fruit, sliced in ½" pieces

8 large strawberries, sliced in half

2 medium pears, cut into ½" pieces

1 large orange, sliced into ½" pieces

1 cup plain, low-fat yogurt

Juice of 1 lime

2 teaspoons fresh mint leaves, finely chopped

1. Arrange cut fruit pieces on 8 wooden skewers, alternating fruit types.

2. In a small bowl, mix yogurt, lime juice, and mint.

3. Serve fruit skewers with yogurt dip.

PER SERVING: Calories: 159 | GI: Low | Carbohydrates: 35g | Protein: 5g | Fat: 2g

Fresh Herbed Yogurt

Herbs and citrus make yogurt taste great. For a different flavor, try using fresh basil leaves and the juice of half a lemon. You may also use other low GI fresh fruits like bananas and apples.

Broiled Herb-Crusted Chicken Tenders

Chicken tenders are always popular with kids, and you can try this for entertaining adults, too. The skewers make the chicken tenders easy and fun for kids to eat with their hands and make these chicken tenders a convenient appetizer for a party.

INGREDIENTS | SERVES 4

1 pound chicken tenders

¼ cup olive oil

2 teaspoons dried thyme

2 teaspoons dried sage

Salt and pepper, to taste

8 skewers (if wooden, soak skewers)

1. Preheat broiler to 400°F. Rinse the chicken tenders and pat dry. Mix the olive oil, herbs, salt, and pepper. Dip the chicken tenders in this mixture.

2. Skewer each piece of herbed chicken tender and broil on a baking sheet for 3 minutes per side. Serve with any of the dipping sauces in this chapter.

PER SERVING: Calories: 170 | GI: Zero | Carbohydrates: 2g | Protein: 4g | Fat: 17g

Pita Toast with Herbs and Cheese

These pita toast snacks are an easy alternative to traditional appetizers.
They work well as after-school snacks for kids and as starters for a cocktail party.

INGREDIENTS | MAKES 4 SNACKS

1 whole-wheat pita

2 tablespoons cream cheese, at room temperature

2 teaspoons Gorgonzola cheese, at room temperature

2 sprigs fresh parsley, minced

2 tablespoons chives, minced

Salt and pepper, to taste

Cut the pitas in fourths and then toast. Using a fork, mix the rest of the ingredients together in a small bowl. Spread on pitas and serve.

PER SERVING: Calories: 77 | GI: Low | Carbohydrates: 9g | Protein: 4g | Fat: 5g

Bagel Chips

You can buy bagel chips in the supermarket, but they are usually
so hard you could break your teeth. Try these instead!

INGREDIENTS | MAKES 12 CHIPS

2 whole-wheat or pumpernickel bagels

Spray bottle of olive oil

Garlic salt and pepper, to taste

Fresh Garlic Rub

For a low-salt option try this: Take a large clove of garlic, cut it in half, and rub the cut side all over the surface of the bagels. Rubbing garlic is a technique that can be used on breads as well as chicken and beef.

1. Thinly slice the bagels crosswise, discarding the tiny ends.

2. Spread the pieces on a baking sheet. Spray with olive oil and sprinkle with garlic salt and pepper.

3. Bake at 350°F for 10 minutes. Serve as crackers.

PER SERVING: Calories: 26 | GI: Low | Carbohydrates: 5g | Protein: 1g | Fat: 0g

Creamy-Crunchy Avocado Dip with Red Onions and Macadamia Nuts

This is one of the best dips you can make.
Try it with bagel chips, pita toast, or even good corn chips.

INGREDIENTS | SERVES 2

1 large ripe avocado, peeled, pit removed

Juice of ½ fresh lime

2 tablespoons red onion, minced

2 tablespoons macadamia nuts, chopped

1 teaspoon Tabasco or other hot red pepper sauce

Salt, to taste

Using a small bowl, mash the avocado and mix in the rest of the ingredients. Serve chilled.

Macadamia Nuts

Macadamia nuts are native to Australia and were introduced to Hawaii, where much of today's macadamia nuts are grown, in the early 1880s. These nuts are a great source of monounsaturated fats, making them a heart-healthy food.

PER SERVING: Calories: 229 | GI: Zero | Carbohydrates: 10g | Protein: 3g | Fat: 22g

Rice Cakes

Serve hot or cold and with a sweet or pungent sauce.

INGREDIENTS | MAKES 4 CAKES

1 cup cooked rice, basmati or arborio

1 egg

1 teaspoon sugar

Cinnamon, to taste (start with ¼ teaspoon)

¼ teaspoon salt, or to taste

¼ cup canola oil

1. Cool the cooked rice. Beat the egg, sugar, cinnamon, and salt together. Mix into the rice.

2. In a frying pan, heat the oil to 350°F and fry cakes until golden. Serve hot or cold.

PER SERVING: Calories: 194 | GI: Moderate | Carbohydrates: 12g | Protein: 2g | Fat: 15g

How to Serve Rice Cakes

These rice cakes are so versatile. Since rice takes on the flavor of the foods around it, the options for serving these cakes are endless. Try pairing them with a baked white fish, such as halibut or cod, with lemon and pepper sauce or sautéed vegetables with soy sauce. Enjoy!

Parmesan Tuilles

These are too tasty and easy to be true!
They make excellent cocktail snacks to go with dry martinis or ginger ale.

INGREDIENTS | MAKES 6 TUILLES

6 tablespoons fresh Parmesan cheese
2 teaspoons canola oil
Sprinkle of paprika

1. Grate the cheese, using a box grater on its coarsest side.

2. Heat the oil in a well-seasoned frying pan or a nonstick pan and drop small mounds of the cheese onto the pan, flattening with the back of a spoon. Fry for 2 minutes per side. Serve hot or cold, garnished with paprika.

PER SERVING: Calories: 36 | GI: Very low | Carbohydrates: 0g | Protein: 2g | Fat: 4g

Black Bean Dip

This is excellent for parties or as a snack and is also very low in fat.

INGREDIENTS | MAKES 2 CUPS

1½ cups canned black beans, drained and rinsed
½ cup Vidalia onion, finely minced
4 cloves garlic, minced
2 teaspoons red hot pepper sauce, or to taste
Juice of 1 lime
½ cup sour cream
½ cup chopped cilantro or parsley
Salt and pepper, to taste

Pulse all ingredients in the food processor or blender. Serve chilled or at room temperature.

PER SERVING: Calories: 283 (18 calories per 1-ounce serving) | GI: Low | Carbohydrates: 39g | Protein: 12g | Fat: 13g

Low-Fat Alternative

Cilantro, onion, lime, and hot pepper sauce increase the flavor intensity of the black beans. Nobody will notice that you used a healthier sour cream. Try substituting non-fat or low-fat sour cream for regular to decrease the saturated fat content.

Homemade Hummus

Garlic lovers can add more garlic to this popular Middle Eastern dip.
You can buy hummus at the store, but this recipe is easy to make and much cheaper.

INGREDIENTS | MAKES 1½ CUPS, SERVES 12

1 15-ounce can chickpeas, drained

2 cloves garlic, chopped, or more to taste

½ small white onion, chopped

1 teaspoon Tabasco or other hot sauce

½ cup fresh flat-leaf parsley, or cilantro, tightly packed

Salt and black pepper, to taste

½ cup olive oil

Blend all ingredients in the food processor or blender. Do not purée—you want a coarse consistency. Serve with bagel chips or warm pita bread.

All-Natural Olive Oil Spray

To make your own olive oil spray, you can buy a clean spray bottle at a hardware store and fill it with olive oil. If using a spray bottle from your house, make sure it has never contained anything that could leave a harmful residue. Use this spray as an alternative to nonstick sprays that don't taste like olive oil.

PER SERVING: Calories: 128 | GI: Low | Carbohydrates: 9g | Protein: 2g | Fat: 9g

Polenta Cubes with Salsa

Polenta cubes are crunchy and good for snacks or as croutons on salads.

INGREDIENTS | MAKES 80 1" CUBES

1 cup yellow cornmeal

3 cups boiling water

1 teaspoon salt

½ cup Parmesan cheese

½ cup chives, finely minced

Nonstick spray, as needed

½ cup canola oil

Green Salsa (see following recipe)

1. Stir the cornmeal in a fine stream into boiling salted water. Cook, stirring for about 20 minutes or until the polenta comes away from the sides of the pan. Add Parmesan cheese and chives. Prepare a 9" × 9" glass baking pan with nonstick spray and spread the polenta in the pan.

2. Chill the polenta. When polenta is firm, turn it out onto waxed paper and cut into 1" cubes.

3. Fry the cubes in canola oil at high heat, turning as the sides brown. Drain on paper towels and serve with salsa.

PER SERVING (PER CUBE): Calories: 19 | GI: Moderate | Carbohydrates: 1g | Protein: 1g | Fat: 1g

Green Salsa

This Mexican classic is delicious in omelets or used as a dip. It's a great alternative to the usual red salsa you find in America. Add more jalapeños for some extra heat.

INGREDIENTS | MAKES 1 CUP

6 tomatillos, chopped, husks discarded

4 cloves garlic, minced

2 jalapeño peppers, cored and chopped, seeds included

½ cup sour cream

½ cup cilantro

Salt, to taste

Place all ingredients in the blender and pulse until coarsely chopped. Rest in refrigerator for 2 hours. Serve chilled.

TIP: *Substitute low-fat sour cream for regular sour cream.*

PER SERVING: Calories: 332 (40 calories per 1-ounce serving) | GI: Very low | Carbohydrates: 24g | Protein: 0g | Fat: 24g

Tomatillo Tutorial

Tomatillos are husked tomatoes that look like green tomatoes when their papery husk is removed. You can find them in most major supermarkets. Choose unblemished tomatillos that fully fill out their husks.

Sour Cream and Gorgonzola Dip for Crudités

Perhaps the healthiest of snacks is a plate of raw veggies and a low-cal dip like this one.

INGREDIENTS | MAKES 1½ CUPS

¾ cup low-fat sour cream

¼ cup Gorgonzola cheese, crumbled

½ teaspoon celery salt

1 teaspoon Tabasco or other hot sauce

2 tablespoons lemon juice

Pulse all ingredients in the food processor or blender; serve chilled with a selection of raw vegetables.

PER SERVING: Calories: 268 (22 calories per 1-ounce serving) | GI: Zero | Carbohydrates: 6g | Protein: 8g | Fat: 24g

Mango Salsa

This is excellent with shrimp, crab legs, or fruit.
Avoid using frozen mango since it tends to be mushy when thawed.

INGREDIENTS | MAKES 1 CUP

1 mango, peeled and diced

¼ cup sweet onion, minced

2 teaspoons cider vinegar

2 jalapeño peppers, cored, seeded, and minced

Juice of ½ lime

2 tablespoons cilantro or parsley, finely chopped

Salt, to taste

Pulse all ingredients in the food processor or blender. Turn into a bowl, chill, and serve.

PER SERVING: Calories: 209 (26 calories per 1-ounce serving) | GI: Low | Carbohydrates: 54g | Protein: 2g | Fat: 0g

Mango Facts

Did you know mangos are the most popular fruit in the world? They are grown in tropical climates and therefore are available to be enjoyed year round. In many countries, mango is eaten both ripe and unripe. The unripe mango is often pickled, seasoned, or made into a sauce and served with a savory meal. Sweet, ripe mangos can be made into juice, smoothies, and fruit salads.

Italian Dressing

Try doubling this recipe and storing in a glass jar.
It will keep for several days and is much better than supermarket dressings.

INGREDIENTS | MAKES 1 CUP
(2 TABLESPOONS PER
SERVING)

⅓ cup balsamic vinegar

½ teaspoon dry mustard

1 teaspoon lemon juice

2 cloves garlic, chopped

1 teaspoon oregano, dried, or 1 tablespoon fresh oregano leaves

Salt and pepper, to taste

½ cup extra-virgin olive oil

Put all but the olive oil into a blender and blend until smooth. Whisk in the oil slowly in a thin stream. Bottle and give it a good shake before serving.

PER SERVING: Calories: 63 | GI: Zero | Carbohydrates: 0g | Protein: 0g | Fat: 7g

French Dressing

This is a great dressing on a crisp green salad.
You can also use it as a marinade for beef, chicken, or pork.

INGREDIENTS | MAKES 1 CUP (2 TABLESPOONS PER SERVING)

⅓ cup red wine vinegar

½ teaspoon Worcestershire sauce

1 clove garlic, chopped

2 tablespoons fresh parsley, chopped

1 teaspoon thyme, dried

1 teaspoon rosemary, dried

Pinch sugar

⅔ cup extra-virgin olive oil

Mix all ingredients except the olive oil in the blender. Slowly add the oil in a thin stream so that the ingredients will emulsify.

PER SERVING: Calories: 77 | GI: Zero | Carbohydrates: 1g | Protein: 0g | Fat: 9g

Balsamic Vinaigrette and Marinade

Because balsamic vinegar is very sweet, it needs a slightly sour counterpoint. In this case, it is lemon juice. It also needs a bit of zip, like pepper or mustard. Use this recipe as a dressing or a marinade.

**INGREDIENTS | MAKES 1 CUP
(2 TABLESPOONS PER
SERVING)**

2 cloves garlic, minced

2 shallots, minced

⅓ cup balsamic vinegar

Juice of ½ lemon

Salt and pepper, to taste

½ teaspoon Dijon-style mustard

½ cup olive oil

Place all but the olive oil in a blender. With the blender running on a medium setting, slowly pour the oil into the jar. Blend until very smooth. Cover and store in the refrigerator for up to 7 days.

PER SERVING: Calories: 76 | GI: Zero | Carbohydrates: 4g | Protein: 0g | Fat: 7g

The Condiment of Kings

Mustard is one of the oldest condiments, having been used for over 3,000 years. The first mustards were made from crushed black or brown mustard seeds mixed with vinegar. In 1856, the creator of Dijon mustard, Jean Naigeon, changed the recipe into what it is today—crushed mustard seeds mixed with sour juice made from unripe grapes.

CHAPTER 7

Sandwiches and Wraps

Sausage and Peppers with Melted Mozzarella Cheese

This classic Italian combination is usually served as a sub or hero.
Try it on thinly sliced whole-wheat bread and use less sausage and peppers.

INGREDIENTS | MAKES 2 SANDWICHES

¼ pound Italian sausage links, cut in 8 pieces

½ cup sweet white onions, thinly sliced

4 thin slices whole-wheat or sourdough bread

4 slices red roasted peppers (jarred is fine)

4 thin slices mozzarella cheese

½ cup shredded napa cabbage or romaine lettuce

1. Fry sausage slices in a nonstick pan over low heat. When brown, drain on paper towels.

2. Add the onions and sizzle over low heat until wilted; reserve.

3. Toast the bread. Place the sausage slices on two pieces of toast. Arrange the onions, peppers, and cheese on top.

4. Place under a hot broiler until the cheese melts. Pile with shredded cabbage or lettuce for crunch.

TIP: *Substitute vegetarian sausage for regular sausage and use low-fat cheese.*

PER SERVING: Calories: 295 | GI: Low | Carbohydrates: 36g | Protein: 25g | Fat: 8g

Baby Eggplant with Tomato

Baby eggplants are great to cook with because they don't take very long to grill or sauté and are never bitter. You can get dark purple, mauve, or white ones, all of which are wonderful. Baby eggplants are tender enough so that you can leave the skins on when you grill or sauté them.

INGREDIENTS | SERVES 2

2 baby eggplants, the size of jumbo eggs, stem ends trimmed, cut crosswise in ¼" slices

2 tablespoons Italian Dressing (see Chapter 6)

2 teaspoons Parmesan cheese

1 tomato, sliced

1 teaspoon basil, dried

1 teaspoon oregano, dried

Salt and pepper, to taste

4 slices whole-wheat bread, toasted

1. Preheat the broiler to 400°F. Place the cut pieces of eggplant in a bowl. Coat with Italian Dressing. Place on a baking sheet, sprinkle with Parmesan cheese, and place under the broiler until golden on both sides.

2. Sprinkle tomato slices with basil, oregano, salt, and pepper.

3. Stack the eggplant and tomato on toast, top with another piece of toast, and serve.

PER SERVING: Calories: 200 | GI: Low | Carbohydrates: 33g | Protein: 10g | Fat: 7g

Sweat Your Eggplant

Eggplant is a member of the nightshade family and is related to tomatoes and potatoes. If eggplant is a little overripe (which happens often with larger eggplant), it will have a bitter taste. To get rid of the bitter taste, place sliced eggplant in a colander and sprinkle with salt. Allow the eggplant to "sweat" for 20 minutes and rinse before using.

Hot and Spicy Pork Meatball Sub

Pork makes excellent meatballs.
Spiked with pepper and barbecue sauce, you have wonderful sandwiches.

INGREDIENTS | MAKES 4 BIG SANDWICHES

1 pound ground pork

Salt and pepper, to taste

¼ teaspoon ground cloves

1 tablespoon Tabasco sauce

2 tablespoons chili sauce

1 egg, well beaten

½ cup fine bread crumbs

½" canola oil in a heavy frying pan

4 hero rolls (whole wheat if possible)

4 teaspoons of your favorite barbecue sauce

½ sweet onion, thinly sliced

1. Mix the pork, salt, pepper, cloves, Tabasco sauce, chili sauce, and egg in a bowl.

2. Form 16 small meatballs and roll them in the bread crumbs. Heat the oil to 350°F and fry meatballs until brown and crisp all over.

3. Drain the meatballs on paper towels. Place on rolls, drizzle with barbecue sauce, and pile with onions.

PER SERVING: Calories: 541 | GI: Low | Carbohydrates: 29g | Protein: 29g | Fat: 34g

How to Scale Down Portion Size

To cut back on calories in this recipe, you can make this serve six people instead of four. Make 18 smaller meatballs instead of 16 larger ones and serve them on 6 rolls. This technique may be especially useful if you are making this as a lunch recipe.

Broiled Swordfish Club

Who says you need three slices of bread to make a club sandwich?
What you do need is two slices of whole-grain bread per sandwich.

INGREDIENTS | MAKES 2 SANDWICHES

4 slices lean bacon or turkey bacon

2 swordfish fillets, about 5 ounces each

2 tablespoons lemon juice

Salt and pepper, to taste

2 teaspoons low-fat mayonnaise

1 teaspoon dried dill, or 2 teaspoons fresh dill weed

4 slices whole-grain bread

8 thin slices cucumber

4 slices fresh tomato

1. Fry the bacon and drain on a paper towel. Sprinkle the fish with lemon juice, salt, and pepper. Place under a hot (450°F) broiler for 3 minutes per side.

2. Mix the mayonnaise and dill. Spread on the bread. Stack the bacon, fish, cucumber, and tomato on two slices of bread. Finish with top slice and cut. Serve with extra cucumber slices on the side.

> **TIP:** *Substitute Canadian bacon or vegetarian "bacon" for regular bacon.*

PER SERVING: Calories: 419 | GI: Low | Carbohydrates: 29g | Protein: 39g | Fat: 18g

Fresh Fish and Seafood Sandwiches

Because items like swordfish, tuna, shrimp, and other seafood cook so quickly, they are ideal for a fast sandwich. During the summer, cook your shrimp the night before and refrigerate it, or you can buy precooked and shelled shrimp.

Grilled Vegetable and Three Cheese Panini

Panini are grilled sandwiches usually stuffed with vegetables, cheese, and grilled meat.
They are grilled in a panini press or in a frying pan with a heavy weight on top to squish them down.
You can use a heavy frying pan or foil-covered brick as the weight!

INGREDIENTS | MAKES 2 SANDWICHES

2 baby eggplants, thinly sliced

½ yellow summer squash, cut in ¼" coins

¼ cup Italian Dressing (see Chapter 6)

1 sweet red bell pepper, cored and seeded

2 teaspoons Parmesan cheese, grated

4 slices Tuscan bread (whole wheat or sourdough)

2 slices Muenster cheese, thinly sliced

2 teaspoons Gorgonzola cheese, crumbled

Oil as needed for panini press or frying pan

1. Brush eggplant and squash with dressing and grill. Grill red pepper, skin side to flame, until it chars. Place red pepper, while still hot, in a plastic bag. Let cool, then rub skin off. Slice into strips. Sprinkle veggies with Parmesan cheese and set aside.

2. Spread both sides of 4 pieces of bread with Italian dressing. Load with vegetables and Muenster and Gorgonzola cheeses.

3. Place panini on lightly oiled frying pan or panini press. If using a frying pan, cover it with a second pan or foil-covered brick. Toast the sandwich on medium heat until very brown. Turn if using a frying pan.

4. Cut sandwiches and serve piping hot.

PER SERVING: Calories: 459 | GI: Low | Carbohydrates: 48g | Protein: 23g | Fat: 24g

Fresh Tuna and Wasabi Mayonnaise Grinder

Wasabi is Japanese horseradish and is very, very spicy.
It is delicious when used wisely!

INGREDIENTS | MAKES 2 SANDWICHES

Salt and pepper, to taste

1 8-ounce fresh tuna steak

10 green beans

Water, as needed

¼ cup mayonnaise

½ teaspoon wasabi powder, or to taste

4 thin slices tomato

Sourdough whole-wheat French bread, cut in 5" lengths and split

1. Salt and pepper the tuna steak. Sear on a nonstick pan over medium flame. Blanch green beans for 3 minutes in boiling water; chop. Mix the mayonnaise and wasabi powder; add the chopped beans.

2. When the tuna is medium rare, about 4 minutes per side, slice it thinly. Stack with the mayonnaise-bean mixture and tomatoes on the bread. Serve immediately.

TIP: *Replace regular mayonnaise with low-fat mayonnaise.*

PER SERVING: Calories: 571 | GI: Low | Carbohydrates: 41g | Protein: 35g | Fat: 30g

Shrimp and Cucumber Tea Sandwich

These are perfect as a lunch or cut into small bites for cocktail snacks.

INGREDIENTS | MAKES 2 SANDWICHES

¼ pound shrimp, cooked

2 tablespoons low-fat cream cheese, at room temperature

2 tablespoons sweet onion, chopped

½ teaspoon dill, dried, or 1 tablespoon fresh dill

4 slices extra-thin whole-wheat bread, crusts trimmed

Salt and pepper, to taste

8 slices cucumber

1. Place the shrimp, cream cheese, onion, and dill in the food processor or blender. Pulse until well mixed, but not puréed.

2. Spread the shrimp mixture on the bread. Sprinkle with salt and pepper and top with cucumber slices. Finish with final slice of bread and cut in diamonds.

PER SERVING: Calories: 164 | GI: Low | Carbohydrates: 16g | Protein: 17g | Fat: 5g

Tea Time

Tea sandwiches are small and dainty in order to stave off hunger until dinner time. Traditionally, tea sandwiches are served on thinly sliced, buttered white bread, lightly spread with a cream cheese or mayonnaise-based mixture and topped with fresh vegetables.

Sautéed Crab Cake and Avocado Wraps

Lots of cooks use surimi (imitation crabmeat) for crab cakes because crabmeat can be expensive. Substituting large cabbage leaves for bread in this recipe keeps the GI down.

INGREDIENTS | MAKES 4 THICK WRAPS

1 10-ounce package imitation crabmeat

4 tablespoons low-fat mayonnaise

1 teaspoon Dijon-style mustard

1 egg

Salt and pepper, to taste

⅛" canola oil, in frying pan

4 large cabbage leaves

Water, as needed

1 avocado, peeled and sliced around pit

4 slices fresh lemon, paper-thin

Extra lemon wedges and parsley sprigs, for garnish

Lettuce-Style Wraps

Green or red cabbage leaves are very sturdy and work well for wraps. You can also try using Boston or butter lettuce, which has large thick leaves that hold up when used for wraps.

1. Lightly mix the crabmeat, mayonnaise, mustard, egg, salt, and pepper. Set a heavy pan over medium heat and coat the bottom with canola oil. Form cakes and sauté until well browned on both sides.

2. Blanch cabbage leaves in boiling water and then shock in cold water to stop cooking.

3. Lay out the cabbage leaves. Use a fork to mash the avocado and dab on the cakes. Roll cabbage leaves to make wraps. Decorate with lemon and place a crab cake on each. Garnish with extra lemon wedges and parsley sprigs.

PER SERVING: Calories: 245 | GI: Low | Carbohydrates: 7g | Protein: 18g | Fat: 17g

Thanksgiving Wraps

You don't have to wait for Turkey Day leftovers to enjoy these!

INGREDIENTS | MAKES 12 SMALL WRAPS

2 cups cooked turkey, diced

1 stalk celery, minced

½ cup red seedless grapes, halved

2 tablespoons red onion, minced

¼ cup dried cranberries

6 tablespoons low-fat mayonnaise

1 teaspoon dried thyme

Salt and pepper, to taste

12 large romaine lettuce leaves

1. Toss all but the lettuce together in a large bowl.

2. Lay out the lettuce leaves, add turkey filling, and roll them up.

PER SERVING: Calories: 89 | GI: Low | Carbohydrates: 3g | Protein: 11g | Fat: 3g

Cranberry Additions

Dried cranberries make a tasty addition to many everyday foods. Add them to cereal, trail mix, oatmeal cookies, chocolate chip cookies, and salads for a sweet and tart surprise.

Melted Gorgonzola and Asparagus in Corn Tortillas

While the creamy melted Gorgonzola cheese in this recipe makes it taste luxurious, these wraps are still full of nice green veggies! Remember that the darker green the vegetable, the more vitamins and minerals it contains.

INGREDIENTS | SERVES 2

1 teaspoon olive oil

1 tablespoon sweet onion, minced

½ of 1 10-ounce box frozen asparagus spears, thawed and chopped

1 ounce Gorgonzola cheese

Black pepper, to taste

Nonstick spray, as needed

2 corn tortillas

1. Heat the olive oil over medium setting. Add onion and asparagus and cook, stirring for 10 minutes. Remove from the heat and add the cheese and pepper.

2. Using a grill or griddle that you've prepared with nonstick spray, toast the tortillas on one side. Turn and spread with the asparagus and cheese mixture. Fold in half and brown lightly on both sides.

PER SERVING: Calories: 154 | GI: Very low | Carbohydrates: 18g | Protein: 9g | Fat: 7g

Grilled Pork and Mango Salsa Sandwich

Perhaps the nicest cut of pork is the tenderloin.
It cooks quickly and pairs well with fruits such as mangos, pineapples, apples, and peaches.

INGREDIENTS | SERVES 4

1 package corn muffin mix

1-pound pork tenderloin, trimmed

2 tablespoons soy sauce

Salt and pepper, to taste

2 tablespoons peanut oil

½ cup Mango Salsa (see Chapter 6)

1. Using the corn muffin mix, follow the directions for corn bread. Bake; cut into 8 squares (2" × 2").

2. Sprinkle the pork tenderloin with soy sauce, salt, and pepper.

3. Heat a heavy frying pan and add the peanut oil. Sauté the pork for 8 minutes per side or until medium, turning frequently. When done, let the pork rest for 8–10 minutes. Slice thinly on a diagonal.

4. Place 2 pieces of corn bread on serving plates. Stack slices of pork on each. Top with mango salsa.

PER SERVING: Calories: 371 | GI: Low to moderate (depending on the thickness of the corn bread) | Carbohydrates: 16g | Protein: 39g | Fat: 17g

Buffalo Mozzarella with Greek Olives and Roasted Red Peppers

Mixing textures enhances flavors—the creaminess of the mozzarella is a nice counterpoint to the salty tang of the olives.

INGREDIENTS | MAKES 12 SMALL SANDWICHES

½ cup Greek olives, pitted and chopped

½ cup jarred red roasted peppers packed in olive oil, chopped

2 tablespoons red wine vinegar

4 ounces buffalo mozzarella, thinly sliced

3 large whole-wheat pitas

Buffalo Mozzarella

Unlike most available mozzarella cheese, which is made from cow's milk, buffalo mozzarella is made from the milk of water buffalo. Since buffalo milk contains far more butterfat than cow's milk, the result is a much creamier cheese that is still slightly elastic and mild like other fresh mozzarella cheese.

1. Mix the chopped olives and red peppers with the vinegar. Push the mozzarella and vegetables into the pita pockets.

2. Place on a baking sheet. Bake at 350°F until golden brown, about 15 minutes.

3. When browned and hot, cut sandwiches in quarters and serve.

PER SERVING: Calories: 58 | GI: Low | Carbohydrates: 11g | Protein: 4g | Fat: 1g

Asian Sesame Lettuce Wraps

Lettuce wraps make for a fun finger food or a light and tasty lunch.

INGREDIENTS | SERVES 4

2 green onions

2 tablespoons fresh gingerroot, grated

2 cloves garlic, minced

1 tablespoon vegetable oil

1 pound ground chicken

½ cup low-sodium soy sauce

1 can water chestnuts, chopped

1 teaspoon red pepper flakes

½ cup fresh cilantro, chopped

1 large head of Boston or butter lettuce

1 tablespoon sesame seeds

Vegan Option

For a vegetarian-friendly lettuce wrap use tofu instead of ground chicken. The tofu will take on the flavor of the soy sauce and ginger. Firm or extra-firm tofu will hold up better in this recipe than soft tofu.

1. Chop green onion and set aside. Peel gingerroot, then grate; mince garlic cloves. Heat the oil in a large pan; add garlic, green onion, and ginger and sauté about 3 minutes.

2. Add ground chicken to the pan and additional oil if needed. Then add soy sauce, water chestnuts, and red pepper flakes. Cook until the chicken is brown and crumbling apart, about 5 minutes.

3. While chicken cooks, clean and chop fresh cilantro. Separate and wash lettuce leaves.

4. When chicken is cooked, add chopped cilantro and sesame seeds immediately. Serve chicken mixture and lettuce leaves in separate bowls.

PER SERVING: Calories: 249 | GI: Very low | Carbohydrates: 10g | Protein: 22g | Fat: 14g

Simple Tuna Salad Sandwich

A tuna sandwich is a quick lunch to pack for a nutritious meal on the go.

INGREDIENTS | SERVES 1

4 ounces chunk light tuna, canned in water

1 teaspoon light mayo

½ teaspoon Dijon mustard

2 tablespoons celery, chopped

2 slices whole-wheat bread

3 leaves romaine lettuce

2 slices tomato

1. Combine tuna, mayo, mustard, and celery in a small bowl.

2. Lightly toast bread. Top bread with tuna salad, lettuce, and tomato to make sandwich.

PER SERVING: Calories: 330 | GI: Low | Carbohydrates: 28g | Protein: 37g | Fat: 8g

Greek Chicken Pita

*This salad has the flavors of a Greek salad with chicken and is stuffed
into a whole-wheat pita for a quick and easy meal.*

INGREDIENTS | SERVES 1

3 ounces chicken breast, thinly sliced

Salt and pepper, to taste

1 tablespoon olive oil

Juice of 1 lemon

½ teaspoon oregano

1 whole-wheat pita

2 tablespoons feta cheese, crumbled

¼ cup cucumber, thinly sliced

¼ cup tomato, chopped

¼ cup romaine lettuce, chopped

1. Season chicken with salt and pepper as desired. Add olive oil to a small pan and sauté chicken slices over medium heat. While cooking, add lemon juice and oregano to chicken. Cook until completely done, about 8 minutes.

2. Toast pita bread. Stuff pita bread with chicken, feta cheese, cucumber, tomato, and romaine.

PER SERVING: Calories: 480 | GI: Moderate | Carbohydrates: 43g | Protein: 30g | Fat: 22g

Grilled Ham and Cheese

Here is a gourmet spin on a favorite comfort food—the grilled cheese sandwich.

INGREDIENTS | SERVES 1

1 teaspoon butter

2 slices whole-wheat bread

3 ounces prosciutto or deli ham

1 slice Gruyère cheese

1 teaspoon Dijon mustard

1. Heat pan and melt butter, spreading melted butter to coat pan.

2. Make sandwich with bread, ham, cheese, and mustard and place into buttered pan.

3. Cook sandwich over medium heat for 2–3 minutes on each side or until cheese melts and the bread is golden brown.

PER SERVING: Calories: 360 | GI: Moderate | Carbohydrates: 25g | Protein: 27g | Fat: 17g

Grilled Chicken Sandwich

Citrus fruit is the perfect marinade. The acids work to tenderize the chicken while adding a fresh and tangy flavor.

INGREDIENTS | SERVES 1

Juice of 1 orange

Juice of 1 lemon

1 teaspoon olive oil

½ teaspoon lemon pepper

Salt, to taste

1 boneless, skinless chicken breast

1 teaspoon butter

1 multigrain roll

1 slice low-fat Swiss cheese

3 leaves romaine lettuce

2 slices tomato

1. Blend orange juice, lemon juice, oil, lemon pepper, and salt in a small dish. Marinate chicken breast in citrus blend, covered and refrigerated, for 4–6 hours or overnight.

2. Grill chicken breast for 10 minutes or until juices run clear and chicken is completely cooked. Meanwhile butter each side of bun and place on the grill, buttered side facing down, to lightly toast.

3. Place grilled chicken breast, cheese, lettuce, and tomato on bun and serve.

PER SERVING: Calories: 420 | GI: Moderate | Carbohydrates: 38g | Protein: 39g | Fat: 13g

Veggie Burrito

One bite of this flavorful burrito is a fiesta in your mouth.

INGREDIENTS | SERVES 1

1 red bell pepper, sliced into thin strips

½ small onion, sliced into thin strips

½ cup mushrooms, sliced

1 small whole-wheat tortilla

½ cup black beans, cooked

2 tablespoons Monterey jack cheese, shredded

¼ cup tomato, chopped

½ tablespoon fresh cilantro, chopped

1. In a medium nonstick pan, sauté bell pepper, onion, and mushroom slices over medium heat.

2. Put tortilla on a large plate. Top tortilla with sautéed vegetables, cooked black beans, cheese, tomato, and cilantro. Roll up tortilla to make a burrito.

PER SERVING: Calories: 405 | GI: Moderate | Carbohydrates: 59g | Protein: 22g | Fat: 11g

Fresh Baja Guacamole

For an extra kick, try adding a serving of Fresh Baja Guacamole (see Chapter 3) to this burrito.

CHAPTER 8

Pasta and Polenta Dishes

Asparagus and Cheese Sauce for Rotini

Asparagus in a cheese sauce with bits of ham and scallions is a terrific seasonal spring dish.

INGREDIENTS | SERVES 4

1 pound rotini pasta

Nonstick spray, as needed

2 tablespoons olive oil

2 cloves garlic, chopped

½ large white onion, chopped

½ pound asparagus, cut in 1" lengths

1 teaspoon thyme, dried

¼ pound smoked ham or prosciutto, chopped

1 cup ricotta (nonfat milk is fine)

1 egg, beaten

½ cup parsley, chopped

4 tablespoons Parmesan cheese, grated

Shocking!

To keep green vegetables green after cooking, shock them in ice-cold water after boiling or blanching. Then give them a quick toss in butter or oil for beautifully green vegetables. This works well with beans, broccoli, asparagus, and other greens.

1. Cook pasta, drain it, and place in a baking dish that you have prepared with nonstick spray.

2. Preheat oven to 350°F. Heat the olive oil and sauté the garlic and onion until softened. Blanch asparagus for 5 minutes in boiling water; add along with thyme and ham to sautéed garlic and onion. Mix and remove from heat.

3. Mix the ricotta, egg, and parsley and combine with asparagus mixture. Gently fold into the rotini in baking dish and sprinkle with Parmesan cheese.

4. Bake for 20 minutes and serve.

PER SERVING: Calories: 633 (including pasta) | GI: Low | Carbohydrates: 90g | Protein: 33g | Fat: 16g

Caper, Egg, and Prosciutto Sauce for Orecchiette

Orecchiette are tiny, ear-shaped pasta. (The Italian word for ear is orecchio.*)*
You could always use spaghetti with this or any other pasta you have on hand.

INGREDIENTS | SERVES 4

1 pound orecchiette

¼ cup olive oil

2 cloves garlic, chopped

¼ cup parsley

1 teaspoon dried oregano, or 2
teaspoons fresh

3 tablespoons capers

⅛ pound prosciutto, shredded

4 eggs, well beaten

4 tablespoons Parmesan cheese, grated

Salt and pepper, to taste

Prosciutto

Prosciutto is a dry-cured ham made by salting a leg of pork and leaving it to cure for about 2 months. After the salting period, the pork is hung in a sunny, breezy place for a time, after which it is moved to an airy room and left to age, often for a year or more.

1. Cook orecchiette according to package directions. While the pasta is cooking, heat the olive oil in a heavy frying pan. Sauté the garlic over medium heat for 5 minutes. Stir in the parsley, oregano, and capers. Remove from the heat.

2. When the pasta is done, drain it and place in a large, warm serving bowl. Toss in the herbs, capers, prosciutto, and garlic mixture. Stir in the beaten eggs, tossing to cook.

3. Sprinkle with Parmesan cheese, and add salt and pepper to taste.

PER SERVING: Calories: 663 (including pasta) | GI: Low | Carbohydrates: 84g | Protein: 26g | Fat: 24g

Grilled Vegetable Sauce for Spaghetti

*Grilled vegetables, brushed with olive oil and herbs,
make an excellent sauce for your favorite pasta.*

INGREDIENTS | SERVES 4

2 baby eggplants, stemmed and sliced in ⅓" coins

1 medium zucchini, stem removed and cut lengthwise in ⅓" pieces

1 yellow bell pepper, cut in quarters

4 medium tomatoes, halved

¼ cup Balsamic Vinaigrette and Marinade (see Chapter 6)

1 pound of your favorite pasta

2 tablespoons extra-virgin olive oil

4 cloves garlic, chopped

8 fresh basil leaves, torn

Salt and pepper, to taste

Garnish of Parmesan cheese

1. Set the grill on high. Brush the vegetables with the balsamic vinaigrette. Grill until just done, about 3 minutes per side. Grill tomatoes on a piece of aluminum foil.

2. Cook the pasta according to package directions. In a large frying pan, heat the olive oil and sauté the garlic over medium heat. Coarsely chop the vegetables and add to the sautéed garlic. Chop the tomatoes and add.

3. Stir in the basil, salt, and pepper. Drain the pasta into a serving bowl and stir in the vegetables. Garnish with extra pepper and plenty of Parmesan cheese.

PER SERVING: Calories: 580 (including pasta) | GI: Low | Carbohydrates: 96g | Protein: 20g | Fat: 13g

Handling Cooked Pasta

Many chefs undercook pasta slightly and add it to the sauce in the pan. This way, the pasta absorbs flavors from the sauce. Remember that if you put pasta into a hot pan of sauce, it will continue to cook—be careful not to overcook and end up with mush!

Spring Green Peas and Ricotta Sauce for Baked Ziti

Mixing ricotta and peas is classic in Italian cuisine. If you don't want to shell fresh peas for this recipe, buy a box of frozen baby peas and enjoy. Baby bells are smaller versions of portobello mushrooms.

INGREDIENTS | SERVES 4

1 pound ziti

10 baby bell mushrooms or Italian brown mushrooms, sliced

6 scallions, chopped

¼ cup olive oil

½ cup frozen baby peas

1½ cups ricotta cheese

1 egg, beaten

Pinch nutmeg

Salt and pepper, to taste

½ cup smoked ham, finely chopped

Nonstick spray, as needed

1 pound raw shrimp, peeled and deveined

¼ cup Parmesan cheese, grated

1. Cook the ziti according to package directions. While the pasta is cooking, sauté the mushrooms and scallions in olive oil for 10 minutes over medium heat. Add the peas and stir, letting them defrost.

2. Preheat oven to 350°F. Remove the pan from the heat and stir in the ricotta, egg, nutmeg, salt, and pepper. Stir in the ham. Drain the pasta and place in a baking dish that you have prepared with nonstick spray. Stir in the cheese mixture.

3. Mix the shrimp into the casserole and sprinkle with Parmesan cheese. Bake for 20 minutes.

PER SERVING: Calories: 752 (including pasta) | GI: Low | Carbohydrates: 92g | Protein: 59g | Fat: 15g

Peppery Red Mussel Sauce for Linguini

*Mussels produce the most delicious broth, so they are great in sauce and soups.
Today, most mussels that you buy commercially are farm-raised and don't have shaggy beards and lots
of sand. Also called mussels fra diavolo, this dish is wonderful for a family dinner or an elegant supper.*

INGREDIENTS | SERVES 4

Water, as needed

1 pound whole-wheat linguini

3 pounds fresh mussels

1 tablespoon unsalted butter

2 cloves garlic, minced

¼ cup sweet onion, chopped

1 teaspoon lemon rind, finely ground

Juice of ½ lemon

½ cup dry white wine

2 cups plum tomatoes (crushed or canned is fine)

Salt, if needed

1 tablespoon red pepper flakes

Fun Fact

Red pepper contains a natural chemical called capsaicin. Scientists have found that eating foods with capsaicin may decrease food intake and promote satiety at meals. Red peppers may be helpful in controlling appetite for those who are trying to lose weight.

1. Set a large pot of salted water on the stove for the pasta. Bring to boil, then add pasta and cook according to package instructions. Scrub the mussels to remove the fibrous hair, or beard, then tap them together and listen for a sharp click. Discard any that sound hollow.

2. Heat the butter in a large soup pot. Sauté the garlic and onion over medium heat. Add the lemon rind and lemon juice after 5 minutes.

3. Stir in the wine, tomatoes, salt (if needed) and pepper flakes. Bring to a boil. Cover and simmer for 10 minutes.

4. Drain the pasta and place in a large serving bowl. Put the mussels into the sauce pot. Return to a boil; as soon as the mussels start to open, use tongs to put them over the pasta. Throw away any mussels that do not open. Pour the sauce over the mussels and pasta.

TIP: *You can substitute olive oil for butter in this recipe.*

PER SERVING: Calories: 581 (including pasta) | GI: Low | Carbohydrates: 94g | Protein: 28g | Fat: 8g

Shrimp and Spinach Sauce for Pasta

This dish makes it easy to get both your vitamins and protein in one dish.
Shrimp cooks quickly, in about 2 minutes, depending on the kind of heat you are using.
In a sauté pan, cook for 1 minute per side; on a hot grill, 30 seconds per side.

INGREDIENTS | SERVES 4

1 pound of your favorite pasta

2 tablespoons olive oil

4 cloves garlic, chopped

Juice of ½ lemon

1 bag baby spinach, chopped

1 pound raw shrimp, peeled and deveined

Pinch nutmeg

½ teaspoon cayenne pepper

Salt, to taste

4 teaspoons Parmesan cheese, grated

Preparing Fresh Shrimp

Why go to all the trouble of peeling and deveining shrimp? The reasons are flavor and texture. The vein you remove is largely harmless but usually contains grit or sand that would ruin your meal. Ready-to-eat shrimp are already deveined, but they have less flavor than fresh shrimp.

1. While the pasta is cooking, heat the olive oil in a large saucepan. Sauté the garlic over medium heat. Add the lemon juice, spinach, shrimp, and seasonings. Stir until the spinach wilts and the shrimp turns pink.

2. Drain the pasta and turn into a serving bowl. Mix in the sauce and sprinkle with Parmesan cheese. Serve immediately.

PER SERVING: Calories: 619 (including pasta) | GI: Low | Carbohydrates: 88g | Protein: 41g | Fat: 11g

Pesto for Angel Hair Pasta

The combination of basil, garlic, pine nuts, and olive oil is classic and delicious. In the old days, Italians used a mortar and pestle to make this uncooked basil sauce. For our purposes, a blender works just as well. Make the sauce in advance and cook the angel hair pasta at the last minute.

INGREDIENTS | SERVES 4, AS A SIDE

½ cup pine nuts (pignoles) (can substitute walnuts)

4 cloves garlic

2 cups basil leaves, stemmed and packed into measuring cup

½ cup Parmesan cheese, grated

½ cup olive oil

Salt and pepper, to taste

1 pound cooked angel hair pasta

1. Spread the pine nuts on a baking sheet and lightly toast under the broiler for about 5 minutes. Be careful not to burn the pine nuts.

2. Place the garlic and pine nuts in blender and blend until chopped. Add the basil and Parmesan a bit at a time, and stream in the olive oil while the blender is running until you have the consistency of coarse cornmeal. Season with salt and pepper. Serve over hot angel hair pasta.

PER SERVING: Calories: 466 (including pasta) | GI: Very low | Carbohydrates: 5g | Protein: 8g | Fat: 50g

Basic Polenta with Butter and Cheese

In some parts of Italy, polenta is used more than pasta! It is simply cornmeal cooked in boiling water until soft and fluffy like mashed potatoes. When polenta is cooled, it stiffens up, making it useful for frying or grilling. This classic can be used instead of pasta or potatoes. Serve as a base for stews, veggies, or pasta sauces.

INGREDIENTS | SERVES 4

3½ cups water

1 teaspoon salt

1 cup yellow cornmeal, coarsely ground

1 tablespoon butter or heart-healthy margarine

2 tablespoons Parmesan or Fontina cheese, grated

Pepper, to taste

Parsley, for garnish

1. Bring the water to a boil. Add salt. Add the cornmeal in a thin stream, stirring constantly. Reduce heat to low; continue to stir for 20 minutes or until the polenta comes away from the pot.

2. Stir in the butter, cheese, and pepper. Garnish with parsley.

PER SERVING: Calories: 68 | GI: Moderate | Carbohydrates: 6g | Protein: 2g | Fat: 4g

Polenta with Broccoli Rabe

Broccoli rabe is a leafy vegetable with florets that resemble those of broccoli.
It packs a wonderful and slightly bitter, acidic punch that contrasts with the mildness of the polenta.

INGREDIENTS | SERVES 4

1 pound broccoli rabe

1 quart boiling, salted water

Cold water, as needed

2 tablespoons olive oil

2 cloves garlic, minced

Juice of ½ lemon

Red pepper flakes, to taste

1 recipe Basic Polenta with Butter and Cheese (see previous recipe)

1. Rinse the broccoli rabe and cut in 1½" pieces, trimming off very bottoms of stems.

2. Drop the broccoli rabe into the boiling water and cook for 5 minutes. Shock in cold water. Drain thoroughly.

3. Heat the olive oil and add garlic; sauté over medium heat for 2–3 minutes; add the lemon juice, pepper flakes, and drained broccoli rabe. Cook and stir until well coated.

4. Serve over hot polenta.

PER SERVING: Calories: 74 | GI: Low | Carbohydrates: 3g | Protein: 1g | Fat: 7g

Sautéed Polenta Patties with Italian Tuna

Try this for lunch on a hot day or supper on a warm night.

INGREDIENTS | SERVES 4

1 recipe Basic Polenta with Butter and Cheese (see Chapter 8)

Nonstick spray, as needed

1 pound green beans

¼ cup mayonnaise

Juice of 1 lemon

¼ cup olive oil

2 cans tuna, drained (imported Italian tuna if you can find it)

Salt and pepper, to taste

1. Chill polenta in an 8" × 10" glass pan that you have prepared with nonstick spray. Cool the polenta until very firm, at least 3 hours in the refrigerator.

2. Blanch the green beans and shock. Drain and reserve. Mix the mayonnaise and lemon juice in a small bowl.

3. Cut four 3" polenta patties out of the pan and sauté in olive oil over medium heat. Place on individual serving plates. Add tuna and green beans. Add salt and pepper to taste.

4. Drizzle with the lemon-mayonnaise mixture and serve.

TIP: *Substitute low-fat mayonnaise for regular mayonnaise.*

PER SERVING: Calories: 333 | GI: Moderate | Carbohydrates: 7g | Protein: 14g | Fat: 29g

White Bean, Tomato, and Zucchini Sauce for Polenta or Pasta

Pasta is made of semolina flour, a carbohydrate that has a lower GI level than polenta. Try to find coarsely ground cornmeal for polenta because it breaks down more slowly.

INGREDIENTS | SERVES 4

1 pound pasta, or 1 recipe Basic Polenta with Butter and Cheese (see Chapter 8)

¼ cup olive oil

3 cloves garlic, minced

1 medium zucchini, trimmed and diced

½ cup sweet onions, chopped

1 tablespoon rosemary leaves, dried, or 2 tablespoons fresh

2 cups tomatoes, crushed or chopped (canned are fine)

1 15-ounce can large white beans, drained and rinsed

1 teaspoon oregano, dried

6 fresh basil leaves, torn

¼ cup beef broth

Salt and pepper, to taste

Garnish of fresh parsley, chopped

1. Cook the pasta or polenta. In a large pan over medium heat, add olive oil and sauté garlic, zucchini, and onions. When softened, add the rest of the ingredients except polenta or pasta and parsley. Cover, reduce heat, and simmer for 15–20 minutes.

2. Spoon sauce over polenta or pasta. Garnish with parsley.

PER SERVING (SAUCE ONLY): Calories: 274 | GI: Low | Carbohydrates: 27g | Protein: 8g | Fat: 14g

Polenta Possibilities

Polenta can be made into different consistencies depending on the purpose you would like it to serve in your meal. Using less water, you can make polenta-like cornbread and grill it, or you can add more water to make thinner polenta that you can serve with sauce, meat, or cheese and treat like pasta.

Sausage and Escarole Sauce for Polenta or Pasta

If you skip the pasta or polenta, you can easily turn this into an excellent soup by adding chicken or beef broth.

INGREDIENTS | SERVES 4

1 recipe Basic Polenta with Butter and Cheese (see Chapter 8), or 1 pound pasta

1 pound Italian sausage, sweet or hot, cut in bite-sized pieces

2 cloves garlic, minced

Olive oil, if needed

¼ cup dry white wine

1 cup Italian plum tomatoes, crushed or chopped (canned are fine)

2 cups escarole, torn into small pieces

1 teaspoon oregano, dried

1 teaspoon thyme, dried

Salt and pepper, to taste

½ cup fresh parsley

½ cup Parmesan or Fontina cheese, grated

1. Prepare the polenta or pasta. In a heavy deep frying pan, fry the sausage over medium heat. If very lean, add some water. Stir in the garlic when the sausage is almost done. If the pan is dry, moisten with a bit of olive oil.

2. Add the rest of the ingredients, with the exception of the cheese. Cover and reduce heat to a simmer. Simmer for 15 minutes or until the escarole wilts. Add cheese immediately before serving.

TIP: *You can substitute vegetarian sausage for regular sausage in this recipe.*

PER SERVING (SAUCE ONLY: Calories: 234 | GI: Zero | Carbohydrates: 6g | Protein: 24g | Fat: 13g

The Endive's Cousin

Escarole is a relative of endive and has loose, wavy leaves. The outer leaves have a much more bitter taste, so use the milder inner leaves for salads. Be sure to wash carefully since escarole traps grit and dirt between its leaves while growing!

Vegetable Lasagna with Buffalo Mozzarella

This dish accomplishes the goal of making both vegetarians and meat eaters pleased with what you serve. This vegetable lasagna will feed a crowd and satisfy any type of guest!

INGREDIENTS | SERVES 10

1 package lasagna

¼ cup olive oil

1 fresh zucchini, cut into thin coins

1 cup broccoli florets, cut into small pieces

1 yellow bell pepper, and diced

½ pint grape tomatoes, cut into halves

6 scallions, chopped

10 fresh basil leaves, torn

¼ cup fresh parsley, chopped

Salt and pepper, to taste

2 pints ricotta cheese

½ cup Parmesan cheese, grated

2 eggs, beaten

Nonstick spray, as needed

2 cups of your favorite pasta sauce

5 ounces buffalo mozzarella

1. While cooking the lasagna noodles (undercook a bit to avoid soggy lasagna), heat the oil in a large saucepan or frying pan over medium flame. Sauté the vegetables for 10 minutes, adding the herbs, salt, and pepper at the end.

2. Preheat oven to 325°F. In a large bowl, mix the ricotta, Parmesan cheese, and eggs. Mix in the vegetables. Prepare a 9" × 13" lasagna pan with nonstick spray.

3. Cover the bottom with sauce and then with strips of cooked lasagna. Spoon the ricotta and vegetable mixture over the pasta. Cover with a second layer of lasagna and repeat until you get to the top of the pan.

4. Spread the final layer of lasagna with sauce. Bake for 35 minutes. Five minutes before serving, dot the top with the mozzarella. When it melts, serve.

PER SERVING: Calories: 414 | GI: Low | Carbohydrates: 44g | Protein: 22g | Fat: 18g

Pumpkin-Filled Ravioli

This is a savory way to make use of wonton wrappers. Serve with butter or chicken gravy.
You can also place the uncooked ravioli on a baking sheet and freeze.
When frozen, place them in a plastic bag and store for an easy supper!

INGREDIENTS | SERVES 4

10 ounces canned pumpkin

1 egg

¼ cup Parmesan cheese, grated

Salt and pepper, to taste

1 teaspoon savory leaves, dried

½ teaspoon sage

2 teaspoons butter, melted

24 wonton wrappers

4 quarts boiling, salted water

1. Using the electric mixer, beat together all the ingredients except the wonton wrappers and water. Lay out the wonton wrappers. Spoon filling on one side of each.

2. Dipping your fingers in cold water, moisten the edges of the wonton wrappers and press together, making sure edges are tightly sealed.

3. Bring a large pot of water to boil. Cook the ravioli until they rise to the surface; serve hot with butter, sauce, or gravy.

TIP: *Substitute olive oil for butter.*

PER SERVING: Calories: 130 | GI: High | Carbohydrates: 36g | Protein: 11g | Fat: 5g

Sicilian Seafood Sauce for Rice or Pasta

Sicily is surrounded by water and populated by seafood lovers.
Fish, shellfish, and southern vegetables are dietary staples of this beautiful Italian island.

INGREDIENTS | SERVES 4

¼ cup olive oil

½ fennel bulb (about ⅔ cup), trimmed and chopped; save tops for garnish

1 red onion, chopped

4 cloves garlic, chopped

¼ cup dry red wine, full bodied, such as Chianti

Pinch sugar

2 sprigs fresh oregano, stripped from stems

10 fresh basil leaves

1 cup clam broth

1 28-ounce can chopped tomatoes

1 lobster in shell (claws, tail, and body), cut in chunks, head discarded

12 littleneck clams

12 mussels

2 squid, about 4" each, cut in rings

12 medium shrimp

1. Heat the olive oil in a large pot. Add the fennel, onion, and garlic and cook until softened, about 15 minutes. Stir in wine, sugar, herbs, clam broth, and tomatoes. Bring to a boil; reduce heat to a simmer. Cover and cook for 1 hour.

2. Return to a boil and add the lobster and clams. After 5 minutes, put the mussels on top. When the mussels begin to open, add the squid and shrimp. Serve as soon as the shrimp turns pink, about 2–3 minutes.

PER SERVING: Calories: 338 | GI: Zero (pasta/rice not included) | Carbohydrates: 17g | Protein: 30g | Fat: 18g

Cooking Seafood in Proper Sequence

It is important to start with the items that take the longest to cook. Lobster and clams take longer than mussels, which take about 6–8 minutes. Shrimp, scallops, and squid cook within 2–3 minutes. If you add the shrimp, scallops, and squid at the same time as the lobster, clams, or mussels, they will be chewy and tough.

Gremolata: Tuscan Garnish

This fabulous garnish is an all-purpose flavor maker! Sprinkle it on soups, pasta, polenta, or rice. It is fabulous over seafood stew.

INGREDIENTS | MAKES ½ CUP

Juice and rind of 1 lemon

2 cloves garlic, chopped

½ cup stemmed, loosely packed parsley

Salt and red pepper flakes, to taste

3 ounces olive oil

Use a blender or mortar and pestle to combine ingredients. Blend all ingredients and spoon lightly over just about anything.

PER SERVING (10 SERVINGS): Calories: 71 | GI: Zero | Carbohydrates: 0g | Protein: 0g | Fat: 8g

Short Ribs of Beef over Polenta

This is an easy, Italian way of making those delicious, meaty spareribs.

INGREDIENTS | SERVES 4

2 pounds short ribs of beef, cut in 4" lengths

2 tablespoons olive oil

1 25-ounce jar tomato marinara sauce

1 recipe Basic Polenta with Butter and Cheese (see Chapter 8)

1 recipe Gremolata: Tuscan Garnish (see previous recipe)

1. Using a large stew pot or frying pan, brown the meaty sides of the short ribs in olive oil. Add the marinara sauce; cover and simmer over very low heat for 2 hours.

2. When the meat is almost falling off the bone, serve over polenta. Serve gremolata on the side as garnish.

PER SERVING: Calories: 263 (without polenta) | GI: Zero | Carbohydrates: 5g | Protein: 6g | Fat: 28g

Asian Noodles with Tofu and Edamame

This Japanese-inspired dish can be enjoyed hot or cold.

INGREDIENTS | SERVES 2

1½ quarts water
2 cups soba noodles
1 carrot, sliced
½ cup edamame, shelled
½ cup snow peas
½ package firm tofu, cubed
½ cup bean sprouts
1 green onion, chopped
2 tablespoons low-sodium soy sauce
1 teaspoon sesame seeds
Black pepper, to taste

1. Bring water to a boil and cook soba noodles until done.

2. Drain noodles, rinse with cold water, and set aside.

3. In a second pot, steam carrots, edamame, snow peas, and tofu for 3 minutes. Drain excess water.

4. Mix together noodles with vegetables and tofu. Add bean sprouts, green onion, and soy sauce. Sprinkle with sesame seeds and pepper as desired.

PER SERVING: Calories: 340 | GI: Low | Carbohydrates: 23g | Protein: 18g | Fat: 7g

Citrus Scallops Pasta

This zesty pasta dish can be made in a hurry for a busy weeknight dinner or savored on a warm summer evening al fresco with a cold glass of iced tea.

INGREDIENTS | SERVES 5

1 16-ounce package whole-wheat spaghetti

3 tablespoons butter

2 tablespoons olive oil

1 teaspoon lemon zest

1¼ pounds sea or bay scallops

Black pepper, to taste

1 head radicchio, shredded

2 cups baby spinach

Juice of 1 lemon

1. Cook spaghetti per package instructions.

2. Melt butter and oil in a medium pan. Add lemon zest, scallops, and pepper to the pan. Cook scallops for 1–2 minutes per side.

3. Mix spaghetti, radicchio, spinach, and lemon juice in a large bowl. Transfer spaghetti to dinner plates and top with scallops and lemon butter.

PER SERVING: Calories: 331 | GI: Low | Carbohydrates: 29g | Protein: 28g | Fat: 12g

Spaghetti and Meatballs

This classic Italian dish is sure to please the entire family.

INGREDIENTS | SERVES 6

½ cup bulgur

1¾ cups water, plus 3 quarts

1 pound lean ground beef

1 onion, chopped

4 cloves garlic, minced

1 teaspoon dried oregano

½ teaspoon black pepper

½ teaspoon salt

1 cup mushrooms, sliced

1 tablespoon dried basil

½ teaspoon crushed red pepper

2 tablespoons balsamic vinegar

¾ cup low-sodium beef broth

1 28-ounce can crushed tomatoes

1 pound whole-wheat spaghetti

Parmesan cheese, grated, for garnish

1. In a medium bowl, mix bulgur with 1½ cups boiling water. Let stand for about 15 minutes.

2. Mix beef, bulgur, onion, 2 garlic cloves, oregano, pepper, and salt. Shape small meatballs and place 1"–2" apart on greased baking pan.

3. Bake at 425°F for 25–30 minutes.

4. In a large pan over high heat, combine mushrooms, 2 garlic cloves, basil, red pepper, balsamic vinegar, and ¼ cup water. Stir often until mushrooms start to brown and water has evaporated. Add ¼ cup beef broth to deglaze the pan and continue stirring, loosening all brown bits from the pan. Once the broth has evaporated, repeat deglazing step twice using ¼ cup beef broth each time. Once mushrooms are browned, add tomatoes to the pan.

5. Cover pan, turn down heat to low, and simmer for 15 minutes. Add meatballs to pan with sauce and simmer an additional 5 minutes.

6. Bring 3 quarts water to boil in a large pot. Add spaghetti and cook, uncovered, about 7–10 minutes. Drain cooked noodles. Return noodles to pot. Add sauce with meatballs. Serve with Parmesan cheese.

PER SERVING: Calories: 523 | GI: Moderate | Carbohydrates: 78g | Protein: 32g | Fat: 12g

Homemade Macaroni and Cheese

This is a grown-up and healthier version of a favorite comfort food.

INGREDIENTS | SERVES 5

2 cups whole-wheat elbow macaroni or penne

2 cups broccoli florets

Nonstick spray, as needed

1 cup low-fat cottage cheese

1 tablespoon Dijon mustard

¼ teaspoon Tabasco sauce

Salt and pepper, to taste

4 ounces sharp Cheddar cheese, shredded

4 ounces part-skim mozzarella cheese, shredded

1. Boil noodles in a large pot for 6 minutes. Add broccoli and cook for 2 more minutes or until the noodles are al dente. Drain, and reserve ½ cup of cooking liquid. Return noodles and broccoli to the pot.

2. Preheat oven to 400°F. Grease medium soufflé dish using cooking spray and set aside.

3. Mix cottage cheese, reserved cooking liquid, mustard, and Tabasco until smooth.

4. Stir cottage cheese mixture into noodles and broccoli, and season with salt and pepper. Mix in Cheddar and mozzarella cheeses.

5. Transfer to the greased dish. Bake for 20 minutes or until cheese is melted and top is golden brown.

PER SERVING: Calories: 336 | GI: Moderate | Carbohydrates: 35g | Protein: 23g | Fat: 13g

CHAPTER 9

Vegetarian

Stuffed Artichokes

These can be prepared in advance and then heated up just before serving. Artichoke hearts are wonderful in salads, and the individual leaves are delicious dipped in hot butter or hollandaise sauce. Remember to remove the choke—it is indigestible and spiny.

INGREDIENTS | SERVES 4 (1 LARGE OR 2 MEDIUM ARTICHOKES PER PERSON)

4 large artichokes

2 quarts water

Juice and rind of ½ lemon

1 teaspoon coriander seeds

2 tablespoons butter or olive oil

1 celery stalk, chopped

¼ cup Vidalia onion, chopped

2 cloves garlic, chopped

1 cup cornbread crumbs or commercial cornbread stuffing

1 teaspoon oregano

Salt and pepper, to taste

⅔ cup vegetable broth to moisten crumbs

4 tablespoons Parmesan cheese (4 teaspoons reserved for topping)

Nonstick spray, as needed

4 teaspoons butter or olive oil for topping

Timesaving Tip

If you are short on time or unable to find nice artichokes at your local grocery store, substitute fresh artichokes with jarred or canned artichokes. Be sure to choose plain chokes that are not marinated, which will work best for this recipe.

1. Using scissors, remove the sharp leaf points of the artichokes and cut off the ends of the stems. Pull off the large outside leaves. Bring 2 quarts water to a boil with the lemon and coriander over high heat. Add the artichokes and return to a boil. Reduce to a simmer and cook artichokes for 15 minutes. Drain and let cool.

2. Heat 2 tablespoons butter or olive oil and add the celery, onion, and garlic. Sauté over medium heat for 10 minutes, or until softened. Add the cornbread crumbs, oregano, salt, pepper, broth, and part of the cheese.

3. Cut the artichokes in halves and remove the chokes. Arrange in a baking dish prepared with nonstick spray. Spoon the stuffing into the areas left by the chokes.

4. Sprinkle with 4 teaspoons cheese and dot with extra 4 tablespoons butter or drizzle with olive oil. At this point, the stuffed artichokes can be covered and refrigerated. When ready to bake, remove wrapping and bake for 30 minutes at 350°F.

TIP: *Substitute olive oil for butter.*

PER SERVING: Calories: 238 | GI: Very low | Carbohydrates: 29g | Protein: 5g | Fat: 13g

Cheese Soufflé

Aside from the cheese you might buy for this, it's also a wonderful way to use up bits of cheese that are in your fridge or left over from a dinner party. Plus, cheese soufflé is really an excellent dish for lunch or supper.

INGREDIENTS | SERVES 2

Butter, as needed, plus 1 teaspoon

¼ cup Parmesan cheese

2 shallots, minced

1 tablespoon flour

Salt and pepper, to taste

⅛ teaspoon nutmeg

⅛ teaspoon cayenne pepper

½ cup 2% milk, warmed

¾ cup Cheddar cheese, grated (you may substitute or add, blue, Gorgonzola, or Gruyère)

3 egg yolks

4 egg whites, beaten stiff

1. Preheat the oven to 375°F. Prepare two, 2-cup individual soufflé dishes by buttering the insides then sprinkling the Parmesan cheese around the bottom and up the sides.

2. Melt the rest of the butter in a pan and mix in the shallots. Cook for 3 minutes, then stir in the flour and seasonings. Cook and stir until well blended. Whisk in the warm milk. Continue to whisk and stir until very thick.

3. Remove from heat and stir in the cheese. Beat the egg yolks and add 1 tablespoon of the hot cheese mixture to the yolks, then whisk in the rest. Fold in the beaten egg whites. Pour into the dishes.

4. Bake for 20 minutes or until brown and puffed. Serve immediately.

> **TIP:** *Substitute nonfat milk for 2% milk and replace butter with olive oil.*

PER SERVING: Calories: 580 | GI: Very low | Carbohydrates: 8g | Protein: 40g | Fat: 42g

Cheese Fondue with Crudités

This is an interactive party dish. Use fresh, raw vegetables such as broccoli, cauliflower, peppers, zucchini, onion wedges, or whatever you like! You can poach the broccoli and cauliflower for easy chewing. Kirsch is a German wine made from cherries.

INGREDIENTS | SERVES 2

1 clove garlic
⅔ cup dry white wine
½ pound Gruyère cheese, grated
1 tablespoon kirsch brandy
⅛ teaspoon nutmeg
Salt and pepper, to taste
A variety of your favorite vegetables

1. Mash the garlic into a paste. In a chafing dish or large flameproof casserole, heat the wine and blend in the garlic.

2. Add the cheese, a handful at a time, stirring constantly. When all of the cheese is melted, stir in the kirsch, nutmeg, salt, and pepper.

3. Serve with individual skewers to spear vegetables and dip in fondue.

PER SERVING: Calories: 537 | GI: Zero | Carbohydrates: 5g | Protein: 24g | Fat: 36g

Mini Veggie Burgers

These are quite good and easy to make.

INGREDIENTS | SERVES 4

1 13-ounce can red kidney beans, drained and rinsed

½ cup dried bread crumbs (more if beans are very wet)

½ cup red onion, chopped

2 tablespoons Worcestershire sauce

2 tablespoons barbecue sauce

1 egg

1 teaspoon oregano, rosemary, thyme, basil, or sage

Salt and pepper, to taste

½ cup brown rice, cooked

2 tablespoons canola oil

1. Pulse all but the rice and canola oil in the food processor or blender. Turn into a bowl.

2. Add brown rice to bean mixture.

3. Form into mini burgers. Heat oil to 300°F and fry burgers until very hot. Serve on rolls or plain.

PER SERVING: Calories: 251 | GI: Very low | Carbohydrates: 34g | Protein: 11g | Fat: 10g

The Praises of Brown Rice

Unlike white rice, which is rice with its outer layers removed, brown rice has lost only the hard outer hull of the grain when it gets to the store. As a result, brown rice contains many more nutrients than its more processed relative. Also, the fiber in brown rice decreases your risk for colon cancer and helps lower cholesterol!

Stuffed Peppers with Rice and Spices

Green peppers are divine, but red, yellow, and orange peppers have more vitamin C.
You can mix leftover veggies in with the rice or lentils for an impromptu supper.
This one is a favorite for a midwinter lunch.

INGREDIENTS | SERVES 2

1 ounce olive oil

¼ cup red onion, finely chopped

1 clove garlic, minced

2 sprigs fresh parsley, minced

1 teaspoon coriander seeds, cracked

Tabasco sauce, to taste

1 teaspoon dried thyme

Salt and pepper, to taste

1 cup cooked basmati rice

2 extra-large sweet red or green bell peppers

Nonstick spray, as needed

2 cups plum tomatoes, drained and puréed

2 tablespoons Parmesan cheese, grated

1. Heat olive oil over medium-low flame. Stir in onions and garlic and sauté for 4 minutes. Add the parsley, coriander, Tabasco, thyme, salt, and pepper. When well mixed, spoon in the rice, stirring to coat with oil, herbs, and spices.

2. Preheat the oven to 350°F. Split the peppers lengthwise and lay them in a baking pan prepared with nonstick spray. Fill the peppers with the rice mixture.

3. Pour the puréed tomatoes over the top. Sprinkle with Parmesan cheese. Bake for 35 minutes.

PER SERVING: Calories: 329 | GI: Very low | Carbohydrates: 41g | Protein: 9g | Fat: 16g

Ratatouille with White Beans

This is a classic French dish of stewed vegetables, often including tomatoes and eggplant, served as an appetizer or side dish. Serving it over beans makes it a bit heartier and very satisfying.

INGREDIENTS | SERVES 2

¼ cup olive oil

2 baby eggplants, chopped

1 onion, sliced

2 cloves garlic, minced

1 small zucchini, chopped

2 medium tomatoes, chopped

1 teaspoon each of dried parsley, thyme, and rosemary; if fresh, 1 tablespoon of each

Salt and pepper, to taste

1 13-ounce can white beans, drained and rinsed

1. Heat the olive oil. Sauté the eggplant, onion, garlic, and zucchini for 5 minutes.

2. Add tomatoes, herbs, salt, and pepper. Cover and simmer for 10 minutes. Warm the beans and serve by pouring vegetables over the beans.

A Provençal Delight

Ratatouille is a versatile vegetable stew that can be served hot (either alone or as a side dish), at room temperature, or even cold as an appetizer on toast or crackers. As an appetizer, it is similar to the Italian tomato, onion, and basil salad called bruschetta.

PER SERVING: Calories: 409 | GI: Very low | Carbohydrates: 59g | Protein: 24g | Fat: 16g

Cold Tomato Soup with Tofu

Tofu is an excellent meat substitute. It's light and filling and absorbs other flavors in a dish. You can blend it and use it instead of yogurt or cream for a creamy look and texture. This is a perfect vegan lunch that you can serve hot or cold.

INGREDIENTS | SERVES 2

6 ounces satin tofu

8 ounces tomato juice

½ cup sweet onion, coarsely chopped

1–2 cloves garlic

½ teaspoon dried oregano

1 teaspoon chili powder

Celery salt and pepper, to taste

1 teaspoon Worcestershire sauce

½ cup crushed ice

Place all ingredients in the blender and purée until smooth. Serve chilled.

PER SERVING: Calories: 35 | GI: Zero | Carbohydrates: 9g | Protein: 1g | Fat: 0g

Broccoli Rabe with Lemon and Cheese

*Broccoli rabe is somewhat bitter and has a real snap to its flavor.
It is wonderful when prepoached in boiling water and then sautéed in oil with a bit of
garlic and lemon juice. Serve this recipe over rice or pasta, or on its own.*

INGREDIENTS | SERVES 4

1 quart water

1 teaspoon salt

½ cup loosely packed broccoli rabe, ends trimmed

2 tablespoons olive oil

2 cloves garlic, chopped

1 tablespoon lemon juice

Salt and pepper, to taste

2 tablespoons Parmesan cheese

1. Bring the water to a boil; add salt and broccoli rabe. Reduce heat and simmer for 6–8 minutes. Drain and shock under cold water and dry on paper towels.

2. Heat olive oil over medium-low heat and sauté the garlic for 5 minutes. Cut the broccoli rabe stems in 2" pieces and add to the garlic and olive oil. Sprinkle with lemon juice, salt, and pepper. Serve with Parmesan cheese.

PER SERVING: Calories: 81 | GI: Zero | Carbohydrates: 2g | Protein: 2g | Fat: 8g

Wild Rice with Walnuts and Apples

This is a wonderful side dish and is very filling.

INGREDIENTS | SERVES 4

2 cups wild rice, cooked to package directions

2 shallots

1 tart apple, peeled, cored, and chopped

¼ cup olive oil

½ cup walnuts, toasted

Salt and pepper, to taste

While the rice is cooking, sauté the shallots and apple in the olive oil over medium heat for 5 minutes. Just before serving, mix all ingredients together.

PER SERVING: Calories: 417 | GI: Very low | Carbohydrates: 31g | Protein: 8g | Fat: 32g

Pizza with Goat Cheese and Vegetables

You can buy pizza dough from almost any supermarket, bakery, or pizza parlor. When you top the pizza with a good-quality sauce, extra veggies, and goat cheese, you have a marvelous lunch or supper.

INGREDIENTS | 8 SLICES

1 pound pizza dough

1 cup tomato sauce from a jar, or your own

1 medium zucchini, thinly sliced

1 small onion, thinly sliced

20 Greek or Italian olives, pitted and sliced

2 teaspoons olive oil

8 ounces goat cheese

1. Preheat oven to 475°F. Roll out the pizza dough to fit a 12" pan or pizza stone. Spread with sauce. Arrange the zucchini over the sauce.

2. Sprinkle with onion and olives and drizzle olive oil over top. Dot the top with cheese and bake for 15 minutes, or until the crust is brown, the cheese melts, and the topping bubbles.

PER SERVING (PER SLICE): Calories: 178 | GI: Low | Carbohydrates: 9g | Protein: 6g | Fat: 13g

Pumpkin Risotto

This is a fine main course or a side dish, depending on what else you are serving.

INGREDIENTS | SERVES 4

1 small pumpkin (about 3 pounds)
1 tablespoon butter or margarine
1 cup basmati rice
4 cups vegetable broth
⅛ teaspoon cloves, ground
1 teaspoon sage, dried; or 4 fresh sage leaves, torn
Salt and pepper, to taste

Rice Texture

The rice you use in risotto should give the dish a creamy texture, but be careful not to overcook—there should also be a firmness to the inside part of the grain of rice.

1. Peel pumpkin and remove the seeds. Dice pumpkin to make 2 cups. Melt the butter or margarine in a large flameproof casserole over medium heat. Add the rice and stir to coat. Mix in the pumpkin.

2. Stirring constantly, slowly pour ½ cup broth into the rice mixture. Stirring, add the cloves, sage, salt, and pepper.

3. When the rice has absorbed the broth, the pot will hiss. Continue to add broth a little at a time, about every 4–5 minutes, until the rice has absorbed all of it. If still dry, add water, as with the broth, a little at a time.

4. Serve hot or at room temperature.

PER SERVING: Calories: 116 | GI: Low | Carbohydrates: 24g | Protein: 2g | Fat: 3g

Lentils with Stewed Vegetables

*This can be served as a main course alongside roasted cauliflower
and brown rice, or as a flavorful side.*

INGREDIENTS | SERVES 4

¼ cup olive oil

1 onion, chopped

1 small piece fresh ginger, peeled and coarsely chopped

5 garlic cloves, chopped

5 cups water

1½ teaspoons curry powder

½ teaspoon ground turmeric

½ teaspoon ground cumin

1 cup lentils

2 carrots, quartered lengthwise, then sliced crosswise

¼ teaspoon crushed red pepper flakes

1 teaspoon salt

1 cup green peas

4 cups fresh spinach

1. Place olive oil in large pot over medium heat. Cook onion, stirring occasionally, until golden brown.

2. In a blender, purée ginger, garlic, and ⅓ cup water. Add purée to cooked onion and continue cooking and stirring until all water is evaporated, about 5 minutes.

3. Turn heat down to low and add curry powder, turmeric, and cumin. Stir in lentils and remaining water and simmer, covered, occasionally stirring, for about 30 minutes.

4. Add carrots, red pepper flakes, and salt and simmer, covered, stirring occasionally, until carrots are tender, about 15 minutes.

5. Stir in peas and spinach and simmer, uncovered, about 20 minutes.

PER SERVING: Calories: 361 | GI: Moderate | Carbohydrates: 43g | Protein: 16g | Fat: 14g

Roasted Green Beans with Pine Nuts

*Dress up your everyday green beans with toasted pine nuts,
crispy prosciutto, and fresh sage.*

INGREDIENTS | SERVES 6

Water, as needed to fill pot

2 pounds green beans, trimmed

Nonstick spray, as needed

2 ounces prosciutto or bacon, thinly sliced

2 teaspoons olive oil

4 cloves garlic, minced

2 teaspoons fresh sage, minced

¼ teaspoon salt

Fresh ground pepper, to taste

¼ cup pine nuts, toasted

1 teaspoon lemon zest

Toasting Nuts and Seeds

Place nuts or seeds in a dry skillet over medium-low heat and cook for 3–5 minutes. Nuts will have a nutty scent and will be slightly browned.

1. Boil water in a large pot. Add green beans to pot and simmer until tender-crisp, about 4 minutes. Drain green beans and set aside.

2. Spray a large pan with cooking spray and place over medium heat. Add prosciutto and cook, stirring, until crisp. Transfer prosciutto to a paper towel to blot excess oil.

3. Add 2 teaspoons oil to the large pan and return to medium heat. Add green beans, garlic, sage, half of the salt, and pepper to the pan. Cook until the green beans begin to slightly brown.

4. Add in the pine nuts, lemon zest, and prosciutto; season with remaining salt and additional pepper.

PER SERVING: Calories: 99 | GI: Low | Carbohydrates: 10g | Protein: 5g | Fat: 5g

Black Beans and Sweet Bell Peppers

This is a simple and delicious meal that can be made ahead of time and thrown in the oven 30 minutes before dinnertime.

INGREDIENTS | SERVES 2

2 large bell peppers

2 tablespoons olive oil

¼ red onion, minced

2 cloves garlic, minced

1½ cups black beans, drained and well rinsed

1 small tomato

1 bunch cilantro, chopped

Salt and pepper, to taste

¼ cup Monterey jack cheese, shredded

1. Slice peppers in half vertically and clean membranes and seeds from insides. Place peppers in a baking dish.

2. Heat oil in a medium pan and sauté onion for 2–3 minutes, until soft and translucent. Add garlic and sauté for 1 minute.

3. Transfer onion and garlic mixture to a large bowl. Add beans, tomato, and cilantro and mix well. Add salt and pepper to season.

4. Stuff each pepper half with the bean mixture. Cover the dish with foil and bake at 400°F for 35 minutes.

5. Carefully take dish from the oven and remove foil. Sprinkle cheese on each pepper and return dish to the oven, uncovered. Cook until cheese is completely melted.

PER SERVING: Calories: 420 | GI: Moderate | Carbohydrates: 45g | Protein: 18g | Fat: 20g

Tofu and Veggie Stir-Fry

Tofu is an excellent source of protein and calcium.
Choose firm tofu, which maintains its shape better in stir-fry dishes.

INGREDIENTS | SERVES 2

1 cup quinoa, uncooked
2 cups water
½ block tofu
Salt and pepper, to taste
1 tablespoon olive oil
1 cup red cabbage, shredded
1 carrot, sliced
1 cup broccoli florets
5 white mushrooms, sliced
Juice of ½ orange
3 tablespoons soy sauce

1. Add quinoa to a small saucepan and pour 2 cups water over it. Bring the pan to a boil, cover, and turn down the heat to a low simmer. Cook for about 15 minutes, then remove from heat.

2. Cut tofu into 1" cubes; season with salt and pepper. Pour olive oil into skillet on medium-high heat. Add tofu and cook for about 5 minutes.

3. Add red cabbage, carrot, broccoli, and mushrooms to the tofu. Stir, and allow to cook for 5 minutes.

4. Add orange juice and soy sauce and stir, allowing excess liquid to evaporate.

5. Put the cooked quinoa in the skillet with the tofu and vegetables. Mix together and add salt and pepper, as needed.

PER SERVING: Calories: 491 | GI: Low | Carbohydrates: 70g | Protein: 24g | Fat: 14g

Mediterranean Chickpea Bake

This flavorful dish can be enjoyed as a side dish or as a main course.

INGREDIENTS | SERVES 4

5 tablespoons olive oil

1 large onion, finely chopped

4 cloves garlic, minced

1 large tomato, chopped

2 teaspoons ground cumin

1 teaspoon paprika

2 large bunches fresh spinach, washed

2 cups chickpeas, cooked

Salt and pepper, to taste

1. Heat olive oil in a pan over medium heat.

2. Fry onion and garlic for 2–3 minutes, until the onion starts to become translucent; then add tomato, cumin, and paprika. Continue cooking for 5 minutes.

3. Add spinach and chickpeas to the pan.

4. Reduce the heat and cover with a lid. Cook, stirring frequently, until the spinach is wilted and the chickpeas are tender. Add salt and pepper to taste.

PER SERVING: Calories: 352 | GI: Low | Carbohydrates: 35g | Protein: 13g | Fat: 20g

Baked Ricotta Cheese Casserole with Hot Peppers and Vegetables

This is a very tasty way to get your children to consume the calcium they need.

INGREDIENTS | SERVES 4

1 tablespoon olive oil

½ cup sweet red onion, chopped

1 medium zucchini, chopped

1 medium carrot, peeled and grated

2 jalapeño peppers, seeded and minced

2 beaten eggs

1 pound ricotta cheese

2 tablespoons Parmesan cheese, grated

1 teaspoon dried oregano

½ cup fresh basil

Salt and pepper, to taste

Nonstick cooking spray, as needed

1 cup tomato sauce

Optional garnishes: 1 tablespoon capers or green peppercorns

1. Heat the olive oil in a nonstick pan. Sauté the vegetables in olive oil for 5 minutes. Preheat the oven to 350°F.

2. Mix the beaten eggs with the cheeses, herbs, salt, and pepper. Stir in the vegetables. Prepare a gratin pan with nonstick spray. Add the cheese and vegetables mixture. Spread top with tomato sauce and bake for 30 minutes. Serve hot, topped with your garnish of choice.

PER SERVING: Calories: 125 | GI: Very low | Carbohydrates: 4g | Protein: 5g | Fat: 11g

Cutting Down on Salt

Ricotta cheese has a naturally high salt content, so you may want to keep that in mind when adding additional salt for flavoring.

Barley Risotto with Mushrooms and Thyme

The perfect risotto takes patience to create, and the savory end result is worth every minute.

INGREDIENTS | SERVES 4

3 12-ounce cans low-sodium vegetable broth

4 teaspoons olive oil

1 cup onion, finely chopped

1 cup pearled barley

1 tablespoon fresh thyme, chopped

½ pound portobello mushrooms, sliced

2 cloves garlic, minced

1 teaspoon Italian seasoning

Salt and pepper, to taste

Time for Thyme

Thyme is included in a French culinary combination of herbs called *bouquet garni* that includes parsley, thyme, and bay leaves. *Bouquet garni* is often used to season soups and stews. Research shows that thyme has antibacterial properties. Thyme acts as a natural food preservative.

1. Boil vegetable broth in a large saucepan. Remove from heat and cover.

2. Place 2 teaspoons olive oil in a large skillet over low heat. Sauté onion in heated oil until soft and translucent.

3. Add barley, thyme, and 2 cups heated broth to pan with onion; bring to a boil. Immediately reduce heat and simmer while continuously stirring until the broth has mostly absorbed, about 5 minutes.

4. Add remaining heated broth to barley mixture ½ cup at a time, allowing broth to absorb before adding additional ½ cups. Continuously stir risotto until done, about 45 minutes.

5. Heat remaining oil in a second large skillet over high heat. Add mushrooms and sauté until slightly browned. Add in garlic and Italian seasoning, reduce heat to medium, cover, and cook until mushrooms are soft.

6. Add risotto to mushrooms, stir to combine, and season with salt and pepper.

PER SERVING: Calories: 262 | GI: Moderate | Carbohydrates: 49g | Protein: 7g | Fat: 5g

Winter Root Vegetable Soufflé

This recipe puts to good use all of the wonderful root vegetables available in the winter months and provides an alternative to simply mashing them with butter.

INGREDIENTS | SERVES 4

½ large Vidalia onion, cut into big chunks

2 carrots, peeled and chopped

2 parsnips, peeled and chopped

2 baby turnips, peeled and cut into pieces

1 teaspoon salt in water for boiling vegetables

4 eggs, separated, whites reserved

1 teaspoon dried sage

2 tablespoons parsley, chopped, fresh only

1 tablespoon flour

½ teaspoon Tabasco sauce, or to taste

½ cup 2% milk

Nonstick spray, as needed

Soufflé Tip

It's okay to have a soufflé flop, especially in the case of cheese and vegetable soufflés. A dessert soufflé should never fall. If, as directed, you start the soufflé with the oven at 400°F and then reduce the temperature, you are more likely to produce a high soufflé!

1. Set oven to 400°F. Place the cleaned vegetables in a pot of cold, salted water and cover. Bring to a boil; reduce heat and simmer until the veggies are very tender when pierced with a fork.

2. Drain the vegetables and cool slightly. Place in the blender and purée. With the blender running on medium speed, add the egg yolks, one at a time. Then add the sage, parsley, flour, Tabasco sauce, and milk. Pour into a bowl.

3. Prepare a 2-quart soufflé dish with nonstick spray. Beat the egg whites until stiff. Fold the egg whites into the purée. Coat a soufflé dish with nonstick spray. Pour into the soufflé dish.

4. Bake the soufflé for 20 minutes at 400°F. Reduce heat to 350°F and bake for 20 minutes more. Don't worry if your soufflé flops just before serving; it will still be light and delicious.

TIP: *You can substitute nonfat milk for 2% milk when making this soufflé.*

PER SERVING: Calories: 200 | GI: High | Carbohydrates: 28g | Protein: 11g | Fat: 6g

Eggplant Soufflé

Smooth and creamy in texture, this is an Indian favorite.
Often the eggplant is simply puréed and spiced—this is more of a fusion dish.

INGREDIENTS | SERVES 4

1 large or 2 medium eggplants
Water, as needed
1 tablespoon peanut oil
2 cloves garlic, minced
1 small white onion, minced
4 eggs, separated
Salt and pepper, to taste
1 teaspoon curry powder, or to taste
Nonstick spray, as needed

1. Wrap the eggplant in aluminum foil packages with 1 teaspoon water added to each. Roast the eggplant at 400°F for 1 hour, or until very soft when pricked with a fork. Cool, cut in half, scoop out flesh, and discard skin.

2. Heat peanut oil and sauté garlic and onion over medium heat until softened, about 8–10 minutes. Mix with eggplant and purée in the food processor or blender until very smooth. Mix in egg yolks and pulse, adding salt, pepper, and curry powder. Place in a 1-quart soufflé dish, prepared with nonstick spray.

3. Preheat oven to 400°F. Beat the egg whites until stiff. Fold into the eggplant mixture. Bake until puffed and golden, about 45 minutes.

PER SERVING: Calories: 126 | GI: Low | Carbohydrates: 13g | Protein: 9g | Fat: 9g

Okra Stuffed with Green Peppercorns

This is a delightful Indian dish. You can make it in advance and warm it up later.
It's a spicy side dish when you are serving rice or curry, and okra is a nice vegetable
alternative if you get sick of the usual broccoli, asparagus, and zucchini.

INGREDIENTS | SERVES 2

6 okra, stemmed

½ cup vegetable broth

3 teaspoons green peppercorns, packed in brine

1 teaspoon butter

1 teaspoon cumin

Salt and pepper, to taste

1. Poach the okra in the vegetable broth until slightly softened, about 4 minutes. Remove from the broth and place on a work surface, reserving broth in the saucepan.

2. Rinse peppercorns and poke them into and down the center of the okra. Return to broth; add butter and cumin. Add salt and pepper to taste. Serve as is or with rice.

TIP: *Replace butter with olive oil or heart-healthy margarine.*

PER SERVING: Calories: 30 | GI: Zero | Carbohydrates: 4g | Protein: 1g | Fat: 2g

CHAPTER 10

Poultry Dishes

Chicken Breasts with Orange Glaze and Oranges

This is an excellent way to cook chicken.
The flavors complement each other and make a delicious meal.

INGREDIENTS | SERVES 2

2 tablespoons marmalade

2 tablespoons orange juice

1 tablespoon soy sauce

1 teaspoon hot pepper sauce

1 teaspoon thyme leaves, dried

1 teaspoon cardamom, ground

1 tablespoon sesame oil

½ pound chicken breast, halved, bone in, skin removed

1 orange, sliced thinly, skin on

1½ cups cooked brown rice

1. Mix the first seven ingredients. Paint on the chicken.

2. Roast the chicken in a 350°F oven, surrounded by orange slices, for 35 minutes. Serve over rice.

PER SERVING (EXCLUDING RICE): Calories: 225 | GI: Low | Carbohydrates: 26g | Protein: 22g | Fat: 6g

Chicken Scallops Stuffed with Spinach and Cheese

This dish is wonderful for entertaining since the stuffing dresses up regular chicken and makes the dish seem more difficult to make than it actually is!

INGREDIENTS | SERVES 2

2¼ pounds chicken breasts, skinless and boneless, pounded thin

2 tablespoons flour

Salt and pepper, to taste

¼ cup spinach soufflé (frozen)

¼ cup ricotta cheese

⅛ teaspoon nutmeg

¼ cup olive oil

Juice of 1 lemon

½ cup chicken broth

1. Sprinkle the pounded chicken breasts with flour, salt, and pepper on both sides.

2. Mix the spinach, cheese, nutmeg, and extra salt and pepper to make the filling. Spread on the chicken breasts. Roll them and secure with a toothpick.

3. Sauté the chicken in olive oil until lightly browned. Add the lemon juice and chicken broth. Cover and simmer for 15–20 minutes.

PER SERVING: Calories: 324 | GI: Low | Carbohydrates: 12g | Protein: 47g | Fat: 12g

Making Scallops

To make chicken or veal scallops, use a rubber-headed hammer (a tool designed for pounding meat), a 5-pound weight, or the side of a heavy metal pan. Place the meat between two doubled sheets of waxed paper, pounding from the inner to outer edges. Pounding thins and tenderizes meat.

Duck Breast with Mushroom Sauce over Wild Rice or Polenta

If you know a mycologist or visit some farmers' markets, you can get wonderful wild mushrooms. Otherwise, use the shiitakes or brown mushrooms available in the supermarket.

INGREDIENTS | SERVES 2

2 duck breasts, boneless, skinless

2 tablespoons flour

Salt and pepper, to taste

½ teaspoon thyme

⅛ teaspoon cayenne pepper

½ teaspoon Chinese five-spice powder

2 tablespoons canola oil

1 tablespoon butter

4 shallots

1 cup wild or exotic mushrooms, cleaned and coarsely chopped

½ cup chicken broth

2 tablespoons apple jack or calvados (French apple brandy)

1 tablespoon fresh rosemary, or 1 teaspoon dried

1 cup wild rice, prepared to package directions

1. Coat the duck breasts in a mixture of flour, salt, pepper, thyme, cayenne, and five-spice powder. Heat the canola oil to medium high and sauté the duck for 4–5 minutes per side to brown.

2. Remove the duck to a warm serving platter.

3. Using the same pan, stir in the butter and shallots. Sauté for 3–4 minutes. Add the mushrooms and toss to coat with butter.

4. Stir in the chicken broth, apple jack or calvados, and rosemary. Return the duck to the pan. Cover and cook for 5 minutes.

5. Serve the duck with mushroom sauce over the wild rice.

TIP: *You can substitute olive oil for butter in this recipe.*

PER SERVING: Calories: 578 | GI: Low | Carbohydrates: 34g | Protein: 48g | Fat: 23g

Chicken Breast with Snap Peas and White Beans

The snap peas and white beans add to the protein in this recipe and provide a shot of energy that will last for hours. Aside from being a convenient one-pot meal, this is a delectable dish!

INGREDIENTS | SERVES 2

½ pound chicken breasts, boneless and skinless

Salt and pepper, to taste

2 cloves garlic, chopped

1 ounce olive oil

10 fresh scallions, chopped

1 cup snap peas, chopped

1 tablespoon fresh rosemary, or 1 teaspoon dried

4 fresh basil leaves, or 1 teaspoon dried

2 tablespoons dry white vermouth

1 cup canned whole tomatoes, drained

1 13-ounce can white beans, drained and rinsed

1 teaspoon red pepper flakes, or to taste

1. Cut the chicken in large chunks; sprinkle with salt and pepper. Sauté the chicken and garlic in the olive oil over medium heat.

2. Add scallions and toss with the snap peas; cook for 4 minutes.

3. Stir in the rest of the ingredients; cover and simmer for 10 minutes and serve.

PER SERVING: Calories: 571 | GI: Very low | Carbohydrates: 44g | Protein: 54g | Fat: 23g

Chicken with Eggplant

*Adding chicken to a typical Asian-inspired eggplant dish
makes for a well-balanced dinner.*

INGREDIENTS | SERVES 4

4 skinless, boneless chicken breasts

1 pound eggplant

2 tablespoons olive oil

2 cloves garlic, minced

1 medium red bell pepper, finely chopped

½ cup water

¼ cup soy sauce

¼ cup red wine vinegar

2 tablespoons agave nectar

2 tablespoons sesame oil

¼ teaspoon crushed red pepper

1. Cut chicken breasts lengthwise into ½"-wide strips. Cut eggplant lengthwise into 1"-wide strips.

2. Heat olive oil in a large pan and cook chicken until well done. Transfer to a bowl and set aside.

3. Return pan to high heat and add eggplant, garlic, bell pepper, and water. Bring to a boil, then reduce heat to medium-low, cover pan, and cook until eggplant is very soft and liquid has evaporated, stirring occasionally.

4. In a small bowl, mix soy sauce, vinegar, agave nectar, and sesame oil. Add cooked chicken, soy sauce mixture, and crushed red pepper to pan with cooked eggplant and bring to boil. Reduce heat to medium and cook, occasionally stirring, for about 5 minutes.

PER SERVING: Calories: 368 | GI: Very low | Carbohydrates: 11g | Protein: 43g | Fat: 16g

Chicken and Vegetable Frittata

*Eggs and chicken make this satisfying meal both
high in protein and a complete one-pot dish.*

INGREDIENTS | SERVES 4

1 teaspoon butter

3 shallots, sliced

2 cloves garlic, minced

Salt and pepper, to taste

8 ounces chicken breast, diced

Nonstick spray, as needed

1 cup broccoli florets

1 cup zucchini, sliced

1 cup yellow squash, sliced

12 asparagus spears, chopped into 1"
pieces

8 eggs

½ cup low-fat milk

¼ cup Parmesan cheese, grated

1. Preheat oven to 350°F. Melt butter in a small pan over medium heat and sauté shallots and garlic until soft, about 3 minutes. Be careful not to burn garlic.

2. Salt and pepper diced chicken breast as desired. Add chicken to pan with shallots and garlic and sauté until chicken is cooked.

3. Grease a round casserole dish. Place all vegetables and chicken with shallots into the greased dish.

4. Whisk together eggs, milk, and Parmesan cheese and pour over contents in the dish.

5. Bake at 350°F for 20–25 minutes, until eggs are set but not brown.

PER SERVING: Calories: 286 | GI: Low | Carbohydrates: 9g | Protein: 32g | Fat: 14g

Poached Mediterranean Chicken with Olives, Tomatoes, and Herbs

Poaching a skinless, boneless chicken breast is a calorie-conscious and practical mode of cooking. The chicken does not dry out as it does when grilled or broiled, and no oil is necessary.

INGREDIENTS | SERVES 2

1 cup low-salt chicken broth

1 large fresh tomato, cored and chopped

4 ounces pearl onions, fresh or frozen

4 to 6 cloves Roasted Garlic (see Chapter 14)

10 spicy black olives, such as Kalamata or Sicilian

10 green olives, pitted (no pimientos)

½ teaspoon oregano leaves, dried, crumbled

1 teaspoon mint leaves, dried, crumbled

4 fresh basil leaves, torn

2 4-ounce chicken breasts, boneless and skinless

Salt and pepper, to taste

½ teaspoon lemon zest

4 sprigs parsley

1. Make the poaching liquid by placing all of the ingredients except for the chicken, salt and pepper, lemon zest, and parsley in a large saucepan. Bring to a boil; reduce heat and simmer for 5 minutes.

2. Add the chicken, salt, and pepper. Simmer for another 8 minutes and add lemon zest. Sprinkle with parsley and serve.

PER SERVING: Calories: 330 | GI: Zero | Carbohydrates: 11g | Protein: 43g | Fat: 12g

Choosing Tomatoes

In season, use vine-ripened tomatoes. Off-season, use quality canned rather than greenhouse tomatoes. Tomatoes should be aromatic; tomatoes with no aroma will have no taste. Avoid tomatoes with leathery, dark patches—this is a sign of blossom-end rot.

Poached Chicken with Pears and Herbs

Any seasonal fresh fruit will make a dish very special. If you have some fruit brandy or eau de vie,
a splash will also add to the flavor. Pears go very well with all poultry.
Try this for a quick treat and double the recipe for company.

INGREDIENTS | SERVES 2

1 ripe pear, peeled, cored, and cut in chunks

2 shallots, minced

½ cup dry white wine

1 teaspoon rosemary, dried, or 1 tablespoon fresh

1 teaspoon thyme, dried, or 1 tablespoon fresh

Salt and pepper, to taste

2½ pounds chicken breasts, boneless and skinless

Prepare the poaching liquid by mixing the first 5 ingredients and bringing to a boil in a saucepan. Salt and pepper the chicken and add to the pan. Simmer slowly for 10 minutes. Serve with pears on top of each piece.

PER SERVING: Calories: 307 | GI: Very low | Carbohydrates: 15g | Protein: 41g | Fat: 9g

Grilled San Francisco–Style Chicken

This is a quick chef's delight. It's excellent,
and everyone at your table will ask "what is in this?"

INGREDIENTS | SERVES 4

1 tablespoon olive oil

1 tablespoon Dijon-style mustard

2 tablespoons raspberry white wine vinegar

1 small chicken, about 2½–3 pounds, cut in quarters

Celery salt and pepper, to taste

Olive oil, as needed

1. Heat grill to 400°F. In a small bowl, mix the olive oil, mustard, and vinegar. Sprinkle the chicken with celery salt and pepper.

2. Paint the skin side of the chicken with the mustard mixture. Spray a few drops of olive oil on the bone side.

3. Grill the chicken, bone side to flame, for 15 minutes. Reduce heat to 325°F; cover and cook for 15 minutes.

PER SERVING: Calories: 95 | GI: Zero | Carbohydrates: 7g | Protein: 40g | Fat: 10g

Braised Chicken with Citrus

Chicken is wonderfully flavored by lemons, oranges, and grapefruits.
Try it, and use the sauce over rice!

INGREDIENTS | SERVES 2

¼ cup orange juice

¼ cup grapefruit juice, fresh or unsweetened

1 tablespoon orange Curaçao, or other liqueur

1 teaspoon savory herb, dried

½ teaspoon lemon zest

1 teaspoon extra-virgin olive oil

½ pound chicken breasts, boneless and skinless, cut in chunks

Salt and pepper, to taste

Make poaching liquid with the first 6 ingredients. Sprinkle the chicken with salt and pepper. Poach for 10 minutes and serve over rice or chilled in a salad.

PER SERVING: Calories: 274 | GI: Very low | Carbohydrates: 7g | Protein: 40g | Fat: 10g

Lemon Chicken

A classic citrus chicken with fresh herbs without being too sour—
the perfect amount of lemon!

INGREDIENTS | SERVES 4–6

⅓ cup lemon juice

2 tablespoons lemon zest

3 cloves garlic, minced

2 tablespoons fresh thyme, chopped

2 tablespoons fresh rosemary, chopped

2 tablespoons olive oil

1 teaspoon salt

1 teaspoon fresh ground black pepper

3 pounds bone-in chicken thighs

1. To make the marinade, combine lemon juice, lemon zest, garlic, thyme, rosemary, olive oil, salt, and pepper in a small bowl. Place chicken in a large bowl and pour marinade on top. Let marinate in the refrigerator for 2 hours.

2. Heat oven to 425°F. Place marinated chicken in one layer in a large baking dish. Spoon leftover marinade over top of chicken.

3. Bake until chicken is completely cooked through, about 50 minutes. The internal temperature will be 175°F.

PER SERVING: Calories: 254 | GI: Very low | Carbohydrates: 4g | Protein: 16g | Fat: 19g

Braised Chicken with White Beans and Kale

This dish is inspired from a traditional Tuscan kale and white bean soup.

INGREDIENTS | SERVES 4

1 pound boneless, skinless chicken breasts

Salt and pepper, to taste

2 tablespoons olive oil

½ onion, chopped

2 cloves garlic, minced

1 large bunch kale, chopped

1 teaspoon crushed red pepper

1 tablespoon fresh rosemary, chopped

1 15-ounce can cannellini beans, drained and rinsed

1 15 ounce can diced tomatoes

1 can low-sodium chicken broth

1. Slice chicken breasts into small pieces. Season chicken with salt and pepper.

2. Heat 2 tablespoons oil in a large pan and sauté onion and garlic for 3–4 minutes. Add chicken and cook an additional 4 minutes.

3. Add kale to the pan with the chicken in batches and cook until wilted. Season with crushed red pepper and rosemary.

4. Add beans, tomatoes, broth, and salt and pepper as desired to the pan; stir and simmer for 10–15 minutes.

PER SERVING: Calories: 367 | GI: Low | Carbohydrates: 35g | Protein: 38g | Fat: 9g

Emerald Kale

Kale, a member of the cabbage family, provides a ton of nutritional value for very little calories. Kale is an excellent source of vitamins A, K, and C and is known for its health-promoting phytonutrients.

Fried Chicken with Cornmeal Crust

Coarsely grated cornmeal makes an excellent crust for fried chicken. Some use corn muffin mix as the coating for chicken, and while that's fine, it's more wholesome to make your own crust.

INGREDIENTS | SERVES 4

4 half-breasts chicken, 4 ounces each, boneless and skinless

½ cup buttermilk

½ cup coarse cornmeal

1 teaspoon baking powder

½ teaspoon salt

Freshly ground pepper, to taste

½" canola or other oil in a deep pan for frying

1. Soak the chicken in buttermilk for 15 minutes. On a piece of waxed paper, mix the cornmeal, baking powder, salt, and pepper. Coat the chicken with the cornmeal mixture.

2. In a large frying pan, heat the oil to 350°F. Fry for 8–10 minutes per side. Drain on paper towels.

PER SERVING: Calories: 265 | GI: Low | Carbohydrates: 9g | Protein: 42g | Fat: 9g

Turkey Meatballs

These baked meatballs turn out delicious and are far less fattening than fried meatballs. Serve with a flavorful sauce such as a tomato artichoke sauce.

INGREDIENTS | SERVES 4 (16 MEATBALLS)

2 slices whole-grain bread

½ cup 2% milk

2 eggs

½ cup chili sauce

½ cup yellow onion, chopped

2 cloves garlic, minced

1 teaspoon oregano, dried

½ teaspoon red pepper flakes

¼ cup Parmesan cheese, finely grated

1 pound ground turkey meat

1 cup fine, dry bread crumbs

1. Mix all but the bread crumbs in the food processor or blender, adding ingredients one by one.

2. Form into balls and roll in bread crumbs. Bake for 35 minutes at 325°F; turn once.

3. Serve with a tomato-based sauce.

TIP: *Substitute nonfat milk for 2% milk.*

PER SERVING: Calories: 476 | GI: Very low | Carbohydrates: 45g | Protein: 35g | Fat: 20g

Stewed Chicken with Vegetables

This is a good old-fashioned way to prepare chicken for the family.

INGREDIENTS | SERVES 4

1 frying chicken, cut up

1 cup chicken stock

16 pearl onions, peeled

2 large carrots, peeled and cut into 1" pieces

2 celery stalks, cut in chunks

2 cloves garlic, peeled, smashed with the side of a knife

1 fennel bulb, trimmed, cut into chunks

4 small bluenose turnips, peeled and cut into chunks

1 teaspoon dried thyme, or 3 teaspoons fresh

1 teaspoon dried rosemary

2 bay leaves

1 cup dry white wine

2 cups chicken broth

Salt and pepper, to taste

In a large stew pot, mix all ingredients. Bring to a boil. Reduce heat to a simmer; cover and cook on very low for 50 minutes. Remove bay leaves and serve with whole-wheat noodles.

PER SERVING: Calories: 421 | GI: Very low | Carbohydrates: 16g | Protein: 39g | Fat: 18g

A Crown of Laurel

Bay leaves, also known as laurel, are originally from the Mediterranean. They have a strong, woody, and somewhat spicy flavor and are usually sold dried in jars in the spice rack section of the grocery store.

Baked Chicken Legs

This is so simple—an everyday baked chicken that requires no fuss or hassle.

INGREDIENTS | SERVES 4–6

6 chicken legs and thighs

2 tablespoons olive oil

2 tablespoons paprika

1½ tablespoons onion powder

1 teaspoon salt

1. Preheat oven to 400°F. Rinse and pat dry chicken. Coat the bottom of a large roasting pan with 1 tablespoon olive oil.

2. Coat chicken pieces lightly with remaining olive oil. Cover chicken evenly with paprika, onion powder, and salt. Place chicken pieces skin-side up inside the pan.

3. Bake chicken at 400°F for 30 minutes, then lower the temperature to 350°F and cook for 10–15 minutes. The internal temperature of the chicken thighs should be 185°F.

PER SERVING: Calories: 355 | GI: Very low | Carbohydrates: 1g | Protein: 28g | Fat: 25g

Chicken Cacciatore

*This classic Italian dish, also called hunter's stew,
is cooked slowly until the chicken is falling off the bone.*

INGREDIENTS | SERVES 4–6

3 tablespoons olive oil

1 whole chicken, cut up

1 cup onion, chopped

1 cup red bell pepper, chopped

3 cloves garlic, minced

2 15-ounce cans stewed tomatoes

¾ cup dry white wine

1 tablespoon Italian seasoning

Salt and pepper, to taste

1 bay leaf

3 tablespoons capers

Timesaving Tip

A recipe like this that contains a good amount of liquid and a longer cooking time at a lower temperature turns out well when made in a slow cooker. The slow-cooker technique requires very little active cooking time.

1. Heat olive oil in a medium pan. Brown chicken thoroughly, about 10 minutes. Remove chicken from pan. Add onion, red bell pepper, and garlic to the hot pan; sauté until onion is tender.

2. Stir in tomatoes, wine, Italian seasoning, salt, pepper, and bay leaf. Add chicken back into the pan with sauce and bring to a boil.

3. Reduce heat to low, cover, and simmer for 40–45 minutes. Stir in capers. Remove bay leaf from the sauce before serving.

PER SERVING: Calories: 464 | GI: Low | Carbohydrates: 14g | Protein: 25g | Fat: 32g

Duck Breasts Sautéed with Rum-Raisin Sauce

This is a different and delectable take on two holiday classics.
Sweet rum-raisin sauce is often used in desserts—this one is not so sweet.

INGREDIENTS | SERVES 4

2 duck breasts, about ½ pound each, skinless and boneless

Salt and pepper, to taste

2 tablespoons all-purpose flour

¼ teaspoon ground nutmeg

¼ teaspoon ground cloves

1 tablespoon extra-virgin olive oil

½ cup chicken broth

2 tablespoons golden rum

½ cup golden raisins (sultanas)

1 teaspoon Wondra quick-blending flour

¼ cup light cream

1. Roll the duck breasts in a mixture of salt, pepper, all-purpose flour, nutmeg, and cloves. Sauté in olive oil over medium heat until brown on both sides. Set aside, covered with aluminum foil on a warm platter.

2. Add chicken broth and rum to the pan the duck was cooked in. Bring to a boil. Add raisins, salt, pepper, and quick-blending flour. Turn the heat down and simmer for 5 minutes. Add cream and pour over duck breasts.

PER SERVING: Calories: 215 | GI: Moderate | Carbohydrates: 18g | Protein: 14g | Fat: 8g

Duck? Delicious!

While most people believe duck meat to be extremely fattening, it is the skin that is the culprit and not the meat of the duck. Duck meat is actually very lean when prepared without the skin and contains large amounts of protein and iron.

Roast Turkey

The signature main course for a holiday meal or a special family dinner.

INGREDIENTS | SERVES 6–8

1 8- to 10-pound turkey

10 cloves garlic, crushed

1 bunch fresh tarragon, chopped

⅓ cup olive oil

Salt and freshly ground black pepper, to taste

1. Heat oven to 450°F. Place turkey breast-side down on a large cutting board and remove the backbone. Turn it over and place it breast-side up in a large roasting pan.

2. Arrange the garlic and tarragon under the turkey and in the crevices of the wings and legs. Drizzle the turkey with olive oil and season with salt and pepper.

3. Roast for 20 minutes, remove from oven, baste turkey with juices, and return to a 400°F oven.

4. Cook until the internal temperature of the turkey is 165°F–170°F on a meat thermometer. Let the turkey rest before carving.

PER SERVING: Calories: 190 | GI: Very low | Carbohydrates: 1g | Protein: 24g | Fat: 10g

Indian Tandoori-Style Chicken

Garam masala is a combination of spices used in most Indian cooking.
A basic recipe contains coriander, cinnamon, cloves, cardamom, and cumin.
Try ½ teaspoon of each as a base, and then make changes to suit your taste.

INGREDIENTS | SERVES 4

4 chicken breast halves, boneless and skinless, pounded thin

1 tablespoon garam masala

2 cloves garlic, mashed

1 cup low-fat yogurt

Asian Markets

Don't be afraid to ask the manager or owner of an Asian market about things that are unfamiliar to you. You'll open yourself to discovering such goodies as premade garam masala, tamarind pulp, lemongrass, and other delicious additions for your cooking.

1. In a large glass pan, marinate the chicken breasts overnight in a mixture of garam masala, garlic, and yogurt.

2. Preheat the oven or grill to 400°F. Broil or grill the chicken for 4 minutes per side. The hot oven recreates the clay oven, or tandoori, used in India to bake meats.

PER SERVING: Calories: 169 | GI: Zero | Carbohydrates: 4g | Protein: 28g | Fat: 6g

Thai Chicken Stew with Vegetables in Coconut Cream

*Asian flavorings can provide so many minimal, yet wonderful,
additions to rather ordinary foods. This chicken stew is spicy and tastes very rich.
It is loaded with vegetables that reduce the GI value of this dish.*

INGREDIENTS | SERVES 4

2 cloves garlic, minced

1" fresh gingerroot, peeled and minced

2 tablespoons peanut oil

2 carrots, shredded

1 cup canned coconut cream

1 cup chicken broth

2 cups napa cabbage, shredded

4 chicken breasts, about 5 ounces each, boneless and skinless, cut into bite-sized pieces

¼ cup soy sauce

2 tablespoons Asian fish sauce

1 teaspoon Thai chili paste (red or green) or red-hot pepper sauce

1 tablespoon sesame oil

½ cup scallions, greens chopped

¼ cup cilantro, chopped

1. Sauté the garlic and ginger in the peanut oil. Add the carrots, coconut cream, and chicken broth and simmer for 10 minutes. Add the cabbage, chicken, and soy sauce and fish sauce.

2. Whisk in the chili paste. Stir in the sesame oil, scallions, and cilantro. Simmer for 20 minutes. Serve over rice.

PER SERVING: Calories: 540 | GI: Low | Carbohydrates: 16g | Protein: 55g | Fat: 35g

Coconut Cream, Coconut Milk, Coconut Juice

Contrary to popular belief, coconut milk is not the liquid found inside a whole coconut (that is called coconut juice). It is made from mixing water with shredded coconut. This mixture is then squeezed through cheesecloth to filter out the coconut pieces. Coconut cream is the same as coconut milk but made with less water and more coconut.

Jerk Chicken

This is a milder take on this typically ultraspicy Caribbean favorite.

INGREDIENTS | SERVES 8

2 pounds chicken pieces

1 small onion, chopped

2 green onions, chopped into large pieces

1 jalapeño pepper, seeds and membranes removed

3 cloves garlic

1 teaspoon black pepper

¾ teaspoon salt

½ teaspoon dried thyme

¼ teaspoon cayenne pepper

1 tablespoon soy sauce

¼ cup lime juice

3 tablespoons cooking oil

Turn Up the Heat!

If you can handle more heat, crank up the spiciness by substituting the jalapeño pepper with 2 chopped habanero peppers with their seeds.

1. Wash chicken and pat dry. Place in a large glass baking dish.

2. In a food processor or blender, combine onion, green onion, jalapeño, and garlic and chop. Add black pepper, salt, thyme, cayenne pepper, soy sauce, lime juice, and oil and process until smooth.

3. Pour mixture over chicken and stir well to coat evenly. Cover with plastic wrap and refrigerate for 12 hours or overnight.

4. Preheat oven to 425°F. Place chicken in one layer in a greased roasting pan. Bake for approximately 50 minutes.

PER SERVING: Calories: 177 | GI: Very low | Carbohydrates: 2g | Protein: 26g | Fat: 7g

Chicken Tagine with Black Olives

*This tantalizing one-pot meal is bursting with spices,
fresh herbs, and Moroccan flavor.*

INGREDIENTS | SERVES 6

4 tablespoons cooking oil

1 large onion, thinly sliced

2 cloves garlic, minced

¼ teaspoon ground cinnamon

1 teaspoon ground ginger

1 teaspoon ground cumin

2 teaspoons cilantro, chopped

½ teaspoon black pepper

Pinch cayenne pepper

Salt, to taste

1 large tomato, chopped

3 cups canned chickpeas, drained and rinsed

½ cup water

1 whole chicken, cut up

1 cup black olives, pitted

1. Add oil to a large pan over medium-high heat; set lid aside. Add onion to hot oil, and cook, stirring occasionally, until tender. Add garlic, spices, black and cayenne pepper, and salt as desired. Cook, continuously stirring, for 1 minute. Add tomato, chickpeas, and water, and bring to boil.

2. Season chicken pieces with salt. Place chicken in sauce, turn down heat to medium-low, cover, and simmer. Cook for 35 minutes. Add olives and continue cooking for 10 additional minutes.

PER SERVING: Calories: 619 | GI: Low | Carbohydrates: 33g | Protein: 30g | Fat: 40g

Skewered Chicken Satay with Baby Eggplants

*This combination of grilled vegetables, chicken, and Asian flavors is delicious
and complemented by the easy-to-make peanut dipping sauce.*

INGREDIENTS | SERVES 4

12 bamboo skewers, soaked in water for 1 hour

1 pound skinless, boneless chicken breast, cut into bite-sized chunks

2 baby eggplants, cut in half lengthwise, unpeeled

¼ cup lemon juice

¼ cup soy sauce

Salt and pepper, to taste

½ cup creamy peanut butter

¼ cup soy sauce

1 tablespoon pineapple juice

1 teaspoon Tabasco sauce

1 head romaine lettuce leaves (save small white hearts for salad)

1. Skewer the chicken and eggplants on separate skewers. Mix the lemon juice, soy sauce, salt, and pepper. Brush the lemon-soy mixture on the eggplant halves first, then the chicken.

2. Set grill on medium or use the broiler on high.

3. Make the peanut dipping sauce by mixing the peanut butter, soy sauce, pineapple juice, and Tabasco. If too thick, add more pineapple juice.

4. Grill the chicken and eggplants for 4–5 minutes per side, turning frequently.

5. Dip skewered chicken and eggplant in peanut dipping sauce to serve. Use the lettuce leaves as wraps to prevent burning your hands or getting sticky.

PER SERVING: Calories: 438 | GI: Very low | Carbohydrates: 11g | Protein: 51g | Fat: 24g

CHAPTER 11

Beef Dishes

Filet Mignon and Roasted Red Pepper Wraps

*When you are cutting calories and carbohydrates but still want loads of flavor,
this is a great way to do it! You will get carbohydrates from the pepper and lettuce.*

INGREDIENTS | SERVES 2

4 large, outside leaves of romaine lettuce

1 tablespoon olive oil

1 sweet onion, such as Vidalia, finely chopped

1 clove garlic, minced

Salt and pepper, to taste

1 8-ounce filet mignon, thinly sliced

4 slices white American cheese

1 teaspoon Worcestershire sauce

½ teaspoon Tabasco sauce, or to taste

2 ounces roasted red pepper, chopped (from a jar is fine)

1. Lay the lettuce out on paper towels. Add the olive oil to the bottom of a medium frying pan; set on medium heat. Sauté the onion and garlic for 1–2 minutes.

2. Sprinkle salt and pepper on the filet mignon and sauté for about 3–4 minutes.

3. Place a piece of cheese on each lettuce leaf; pile on onions, garlic, and sliced filet mignon. Sprinkle with Worcestershire sauce and Tabasco sauce. Add roasted red peppers. Wrap and serve.

PER SERVING: Calories: 415 | GI: Zero | Carbohydrates: 7g | Protein: 44g | Fat: 31g

London Broil with Grilled Vegetables

London broil is a lot cheaper than filet mignon and is still very tasty. You can use meat tenderizer on it or marinate to add to the flavor. This meal is perfect when cooked on the grill with the veggies on skewers.

INGREDIENTS | SERVES 2

2 tablespoons olive oil

1 teaspoon red wine vinegar

1 tablespoon steak sauce

1 teaspoon salt, or to taste

1 teaspoon red pepper flakes, or to taste

1 zucchini, cut into 1" chunks

1 orange or yellow pepper, seeded and cored, cut into quarters

2 sweet onions, cut into thick chunks

4 cherry tomatoes

½ pound London broil, cut into chunks

4 wooden skewers, presoaked for 30 minutes

1. In a small bowl, mix the olive oil, vinegar, steak sauce, and seasonings and set aside. Skewer the vegetables.

2. Brush the vegetables with the dressing. Toss the London broil in the rest of the dressing to coat and skewer.

3. Heat grill to 350°F and roast the vegetables and meat to the desired level of doneness.

PER SERVING: Calories: 354 | GI: Very low | Carbohydrates: 26g | Protein: 39g | Fat: 12g

Keep Your Eye on the Beef

Beef is high-quality protein, but beware when you eat too much of it or have it with rich sauces, the caloric count skyrockets.

London Broil with Onions and Sweet Potato Sticks

This will give you a real energy boost!
To get the maximum energy out of this recipe, eat slowly and enjoy a smaller portion.

INGREDIENTS | SERVES 2

1 tablespoon olive oil

½ pound London broil, diced

Salt and pepper, to taste

Steak seasoning, to taste

½ cup sweet onion, chopped

Hot red pepper flakes, to taste

1 teaspoon Worcestershire sauce

2 tablespoons salsa

2 large sweet red bell peppers, cut lengthwise, cored and seeded

1 recipe Baked Sweet Potato Sticks (see Chapter 15)

What Is London Broil?

Surprisingly, London broil is not actually a cut of beef but a cooking method. Although many grocery stores and butchers may have a very lean piece of meat labeled as a London broil, it is likely to be a top round roast or top round steak.

1. Heat olive oil over medium flame in a frying pan. Season the steak with salt, pepper, and steak seasoning. Add steak and onions to the pan and sauté until the steak reaches the desired level of doneness. Use a meat thermometer to test the internal temperature of the meat. At 130°F, the steak will be medium-rare.

2. Sprinkle steak with hot pepper flakes and Worcestershire sauce. Mix in salsa and stuff the red peppers with the mixture.

3. Serve with the Baked Sweet Potato Sticks on the side.

PER SERVING: Calories: 384 (with baked sweet potato sticks) | GI: Moderate | Carbohydrates: 26g | Protein: 38g | Fat: 15g

Sirloin Steak and Tomato Salad on Scandinavian Flatbread

Scandinavian flatbread, which you can find at most supermarkets, makes a wonderful, crunchy base for lots of good things to eat. It's flavored with rye and can support strong flavors.

INGREDIENTS | SERVES 2

½ pound lean, boneless sirloin steak, thinly sliced

2 tablespoons plus 2 teaspoons French Dressing (see Chapter 6)

Salt and pepper, to taste

Nonstick spray, as needed, or 1 teaspoon olive oil

4 flatbreads

4 slices ripe tomato, halved

1. Marinate the steak in 2 tablespoons dressing for 20 minutes. Sprinkle with salt and pepper. Heat a frying pan to medium-high and use nonstick spray or oil.

2. Quickly sear the slices of steak on both sides for about 3–4 minutes and pile on the flatbread. Add tomato slices and a bit more French Dressing. Serve.

PER SERVING: Calories: 469 | GI: Low | Carbohydrates: 31g | Protein: 41g | Fat: 24g

Filet Mignon

When you need a protein fix, mix in some carbohydrates, like the mushrooms in this recipe, to boost your energy and brainpower.

INGREDIENTS | SERVES 2

1 8-ounce filet mignon

Salt and pepper, to taste

Nonstick spray, as needed

½ cup white button mushrooms, chopped

2 ounces dry red wine

2 ounces beef broth

Optional: 2 teaspoons Aioli (see Chapter 14)

1. Sprinkle the filet mignon with salt and pepper. Heat a heavy frying pan prepared with nonstick spray over medium-high flame.

2. Sear the filet mignon quickly on both sides. Stir in the mushrooms. Remove beef when at desired level of doneness. Add the liquids and bring to a boil. Pour the sauce over the beef. Serve hot with optional Aioli.

PER SERVING: Calories: 266 | GI: Zero | Carbohydrates: 3g | Protein: 33g | Fat: 11g

Beef Tenderloin with Chimichurri

*This is simple to make for an easy weeknight meal
or perfect for a sophisticated gourmet dinner party.*

INGREDIENTS | SERVES 2

1 cup parsley

3 cloves garlic

¼ cup capers, drained

2 tablespoons red wine vinegar

1 teaspoon Dijon mustard

2 tablespoons olive oil

Salt and pepper, to taste

2 5-ounce beef tenderloins

1. Blend together parsley, garlic, capers, vinegar, mustard, and oil. Season with salt and pepper as desired.

2. Grill steaks to medium-rare. Serve with chimichurri.

PER SERVING: Calories: 435 | GI: Very low | Carbohydrates: 4g | Protein: 37g | Fat: 30g

Grilled Pepper Steak

This recipe combines steak with all the right carbohydrates, such as those found in onions, peppers, mushrooms, and tomatoes. You can stack the steak and veggies on a bun or serve on a bed of lettuce.

INGREDIENTS | SERVES 2

2 cubed steaks (also called sandwich steaks)

Salt and pepper, to taste

1 teaspoon steak sauce, such as A.1. or Lea & Perrins

4 frying peppers, halved, (the thin-skinned, light green variety)

1 large portobello mushroom

2 red onions, thickly sliced

3 tablespoons Italian Dressing (see Chapter 6)

2 cups lettuce

1. Set the grill on high. Sprinkle the steaks with salt and pepper and spread with steak sauce.

2. Brush the peppers, mushroom, and onion slices with Italian dressing. Grill steaks for about 4 minutes per side for medium and grill the vegetables until they are slightly charred.

3. Place the steaks on beds of lettuce and pile the veggies on top. Slice the mushroom and arrange with the steaks, peppers, and onions.

PER SERVING: Calories: 284 | GI: Zero | Carbohydrates: 9g | Protein: 28g | Fat: 15g

Black Bean Chili with Beef and Corn

This will give your family a meal with real punch, staying power, and nutrition.

INGREDIENTS | SERVES 4

2 tablespoons olive or other cooking oil

½ pound ground beef

1 large red onion, chopped

2 cloves garlic, minced

1 large sweet red bell pepper, chopped

1 small hot pepper, cored, seeded, and minced

1 teaspoon ground cumin

1 teaspoon dried cilantro or parsley (fresh is better)

8 ounces frozen corn

2 13-ounce cans black beans, drained and rinsed

1 cup crushed tomatoes (canned is fine)

Salt and pepper, to taste

Juice of ½ lime

2 ounces Monterey jack cheese, shredded

1. In a large, ovenproof casserole, heat the oil over medium flame. Brown the beef. Move to one side of the casserole dish and sauté the onion, garlic, and peppers for 5 minutes. Stir in the cumin and cilantro and mix well.

2. Preheat oven to 340°F. Stir in the corn, black beans, tomatoes, salt, and pepper. Sprinkle with lime juice. Stir to mix.

3. Spread the top with cheese and bake for 30 minutes, or until hot and bubbling. Serve with corn bread or tortillas.

PER SERVING: Calories: 429 | GI: Low | Carbohydrates: 69g | Protein: 23g | Fat: 13g

Legumes

Beans are legumes, as are other foods such as lentils, peas, soybeans, and peanuts. Not only are legumes good for farmers to produce because their roots produce nitrogen, which fertilizes land, but they are delicious and full of healthy protein for you!

Pot Roast with Vegetables and Gravy

As a family dinner, this can't be beat. The leftovers can be reheated with gravy and served over noodles or toast for a quick lunch or supper.

INGREDIENTS | SERVES 6

3 pounds beef bottom round roast, trimmed of fat

2 tablespoons canola oil

4 sweet medium onions, chopped

4 cloves garlic, chopped

4 carrots, peeled and chopped

4 celery stalks, chopped

8 small bluenose turnips, peeled and chopped

1" gingerroot, peeled and minced

1 13-ounce can beef broth

½ cup dry red wine

Salt and pepper, to taste

Wondra flour, to thicken

1. Brown the beef in oil at medium-high heat in a large pot and set aside; add the onion, garlic, carrots, celery, turnips, and gingerroot to the pot and cook, stirring until wilted. Return the beef to the pot and add the rest of the ingredients. Cover and cook over very low heat for 3 hours.

2. To serve, slice the beef across, not with, the grain. Serve surrounded by vegetables and place the gravy on the side or over the top.

> **TIP:** You can lower the fat of this recipe by reducing the amount of meat you use and by browning the meat in cooking spray instead of oil.

PER SERVING: Calories: 590 | GI: Very low | Carbohydrates: 24g | Protein: 67g | Fat: 24g

Corned Beef and Cabbage

The slow cooker is the secret cooking technique of the busy home cook. It requires little attention, and the meat will come out tender and juicy.

INGREDIENTS | SERVES 10

3 pounds corned beef brisket

3 carrots, cut into 3" pieces

3 onions, quartered

1 cup water

½ small head cabbage, cut into wedges

1. Place beef, carrots, onions, and water in a slow cooker. Cover and cook on low for 8–10 hours.

2. Add cabbage to the slow cooker; be sure to submerge the cabbage in liquid. Turn the heat up to high, cover, and cook for up to 2–3 hours.

PER SERVING: Calories: 300 | GI: Very low | Carbohydrates: 7g | Protein: 21g | Fat: 20g

Beef Brisket with Onions and Mushrooms

A roast so packed with flavor it will melt in your mouth.

INGREDIENTS | SERVES 4

4 cloves garlic

½ teaspoon salt, plus more to taste

4 tablespoons olive oil

½ bunch rosemary, chopped

1 pound beef brisket

Freshly ground pepper, to taste

3 large onions, quartered

3 cups white mushrooms, sliced

3 celery stalks, cut into large chunks

2 cups dry red cooking wine

1 16-ounce can whole tomatoes, chopped

2 bay leaves

Kitchen Gadgets

The mortar and pestle was originally used in pharmacies to crush ingredients together to make medicines. In the culinary world, the mortar and pestle is a very useful tool for crushing seeds and nuts and making guacamole, pesto, and garlic paste.

1. Preheat oven to 325°F.

2. Using a mortar and pestle or the back of a spoon and a bowl, mash together the garlic, ½ teaspoon salt, 2 tablespoons oil, and chopped rosemary leaves to make a paste.

3. Season the brisket with salt and pepper. Heat remaining olive oil in a large pan, place brisket in the pan, and sear over medium-high heat to make a dark crust on both sides. Place in a large roasting pan and spread the rosemary paste on the brisket. Place the onion, mushrooms, and celery around the brisket in the pan. Pour wine and tomatoes over top and toss in the bay leaves.

4. Tightly cover the pan with foil and place in the oven. Bake for about 4 hours, basting with pan juices every 30 minutes, until the beef is very tender.

5. Let the brisket rest for 15 minutes before slicing it across the grain at a slight diagonal. Remove bay leaves before serving.

PER SERVING: Calories: 633 | GI: Low | Carbohydrates: 26g | Protein: 25g | Fat: 39g

Filet Mignon Strips with Exotic Mushrooms

This dish gives you both fat and protein with the steak.
To add important veggies and fiber, check out the suggested sauces.

INGREDIENTS | SERVES 2

2 teaspoons butter

⅔ pound filet mignon, cut into strips

Salt and pepper, to taste

6 shiitake mushrooms, trimmed and chopped

¼ cup beef broth

2 tablespoons brandy or cognac

1 tablespoon green peppercorns

1. In a hot, nonstick pan, melt 1 teaspoon butter over medium-high flame. Sprinkle the steak strips with salt and pepper.

2. Sauté the filet mignon to desired doneness, about 1 minute per side for rare to medium. Remove the filet mignon strips to warm plates.

3. Using the pan in which you sautéed the filet mignon, sauté mushrooms with 1 teaspoon butter until softened.

4. Add the beef broth to the pan and reduce heat. Simmer for 2 minutes; add brandy or cognac and peppercorns, stirring to get any brown bits off the pan. Pour Fresh Tomato Sauce for Steak or Chicken (see Chapter 14) over the filet mignon. Add Sour Cream Chive Sauce (see Chapter 14) if desired.

> **TIP:** Substitute olive oil for butter in this recipe to reduce the amount of calories and fat.

PER SERVING: Calories: 359 | GI: Zero | Carbohydrates: 0g | Protein: 44g | Fat: 11g

Ginger Beef and Napa Cabbage

This stir-fry delivers the perfect balance of sweet, spicy, and savory.

INGREDIENTS | SERVES 4

3 tablespoons soy sauce

2 cloves garlic, minced

1 tablespoon fresh ginger, minced

1 teaspoon agave nectar

½ teaspoon crushed red pepper flakes

1 pound beef tenderloin or sirloin steak

1 cup beef broth

2 teaspoons cornstarch

2 tablespoons peanut oil

1 large onion, thinly sliced

½ head napa cabbage, shredded

3 green onions, sliced

1. Combine soy sauce, garlic, ginger, agave nectar, and red pepper flakes in a small bowl. Slice beef into ¼"-thick strips. Toss beef in soy-ginger sauce. Cover, and place in refrigerator for at least 30 minutes to marinate.

2. Mix broth and cornstarch and set aside.

3. Heat half the oil in a large pan over medium heat. Add onion to the pan and cook for 5 minutes until tender and slightly brown. Remove from heat.

4. Heat remaining oil over medium-high heat. Add beef and cabbage to the pan and stir-fry for 5 minutes or until beef is only slightly pink in the center and cabbage is tender. Add cooked onion and the broth to the pan. Cook for about 2 minutes, until sauce boils. Reduce heat to low and allow sauce to thicken.

5. Garnish with green onion before serving.

PER SERVING: Calories: 446 | GI: Low | Carbohydrates: 15g | Protein: 25g | Fat: 32g

Greek Meatballs

Buckwheat instead of bread crumbs is used to keep these meatballs flavorful but still maintain a low glycemic value.

INGREDIENTS | SERVES 10

1 cup buckwheat, cooked

2 pounds lean ground beef

1 onion, minced

4 cloves garlic, minced

2 tablespoons Italian seasoning

1 bunch fresh mint leaves, chopped

2 teaspoons white vinegar

2 eggs, beaten

Salt and ground pepper, to taste

½ cup olive oil

Cucumber Raita

Greek Meatballs taste great with cucumber raita. Try these meatballs with the recipe for Cucumber Raita (see Chapter 4).

1. Mix buckwheat, beef, onion, garlic, Italian seasoning, mint, vinegar, eggs, salt, and pepper in a bowl. Using your fingers, roll the mixture into meatballs.

2. Heat the oil in a medium pan over medium-high heat. Fry the meatballs in the oil in batches. Use a slotted spoon to move the balls in the oil to brown all sides.

3. Place cooked meatballs on a paper towel to drain.

4. If meatballs remain raw in the center, place on a baking sheet and into a 325°F oven for 15–20 minutes.

PER SERVING: Calories: 210 | GI: Very low | Carbohydrates: 6g | Protein: 21g | Fat: 11g

Beef with Bell Peppers

Choose a variety of red, yellow, orange, and green bell peppers to bring vibrant color to this one-pot dinner.

INGREDIENTS | SERVES 4

1 pound lean beef

4 bell peppers, membranes and seeds removed, chopped

3 cloves garlic, minced

Juice of 2 lemons

1 can chickpeas, drained

4 stalks celery, chopped

3 large shallots, sliced

Salt and pepper, to taste

1. Preheat oven to 350°F.

2. Cut beef into cubes. Place all ingredients in a casserole dish and bake for 30 minutes.

PER SERVING: Calories: 358 | GI: Low | Carbohydrates: 31g | Protein: 31g | Fat: 13g

Steak and Mushroom Kabobs

These meaty, juicy kabobs are a hit at summer barbecues.
They can also be cooked indoors on a well-seasoned grill pan.

INGREDIENTS | SERVES 3

1 pound sirloin steak
3 tablespoons olive oil
¼ cup balsamic vinegar
1 tablespoon Worcestershire sauce
½ teaspoon salt
2 cloves garlic, minced
Freshly ground pepper, to taste
½ pound large white mushrooms

1. Cut steak into 1½" cubes.

2. Combine oil, vinegar, Worcestershire sauce, salt, garlic, and pepper to make a marinade.

3. Wash mushrooms and cut in half. Place steak and mushrooms in shallow bowl with marinade and place in refrigerator for 1–2 hours.

4. Place mushrooms and steak cubes on separate wooden or metal skewers. Grill 4 minutes per side for medium-rare steak. You may need additional cooking time for mushrooms.

PER SERVING: Calories: 321 | GI: Low | Carbohydrates: 16g | Protein: 25g | Fat: 17g

Beef and Broccoli Stir-Fry

*Simple everyday ingredients can be transformed
into an exotic Asian dish such as this one.*

INGREDIENTS | SERVES 4

¾ pound sirloin beef, sliced into ½"-thick pieces

Salt and pepper, to taste

1½ tablespoons cornstarch

3 tablespoons peanut oil

1 teaspoon fresh ginger, minced

½ pound broccoli florets

3 cloves garlic

¼ cup soy sauce

Juice of 1 large orange

¼ cup water

½ teaspoon crushed red pepper

1. Season beef with salt and pepper. Coat beef with cornstarch.

2. Heat 2 tablespoons of oil in a wok over medium-high heat, then stir-fry beef and ginger for 1–2 minutes. Transfer beef to a bowl, cover, and set aside.

3. Add remaining oil to the hot wok. Add broccoli and garlic and stir-fry for 3–4 minutes, until broccoli is tender. Take care not to burn garlic.

4. Pour soy sauce, orange juice, water, and red pepper into the wok with the broccoli and bring to a boil. Return the cooked beef to the wok. Stir until sauce thickens, about 2–3 minutes.

PER SERVING: Calories: 290 | GI: Low | Carbohydrates: 12g | Protein: 21g | Fat: 18g

Boeuf Bourguignon

A well-known classic French beef stew.

INGREDIENTS | SERVES 6–8

2 pounds stewing beef, cubed

Salt and pepper, to taste

1 tablespoon olive oil

3 cloves garlic, minced

3 onions, quartered

2 cups red wine

¾ pound carrots, sliced

¾ pound white mushrooms, sliced

1 bunch fresh rosemary, chopped

1 bunch fresh thyme, chopped

Water, as needed

1. Cut beef into ½" cubes; season with salt and pepper.

2. Add olive oil to a large pan over medium heat. Place beef in the pan to brown on the outside. Add garlic and onions to the pan and cook until tender. Add red wine, bring to a boil, and then simmer.

3. Add carrots, mushrooms, and herbs to the pan. Add a few cups of water, as needed, to increase volume of liquid and keep the stew's sauce from cooking down. Cook for 3 hours, occasionally stirring.

PER SERVING: Calories: 383 | GI: Low | Carbohydrates: 14g | Protein: 21g | Fat: 25g

Whole Roast Filet Mignon with Mustard Cream Sauce (Hot)

Filet mignon is equally good served hot, cold, or at room temperature.
If you are serving buffet-style, go for room temperature.

INGREDIENTS | SERVES 14

Salt and pepper, to taste

2 cloves minced garlic, mashed in a press

1 5-pound filet mignon, fat and skin removed

¼ cup dry red wine

½ cup beef broth

10 tiny new potatoes, skin on, cut into halves

15 baby carrots

25 pearl onions

Mustard Cream Sauce (Hot) (see Chapter 14)

Meat Temperatures

Remember that meat cooked in the oven, on the grill, or in a sauté pan continues to rise another 5-plus degrees after it is removed from the heat source. So if overcooking has been a problem, take your meat off the heat sooner, or 5 degrees short of the doneness temperature desired.

1. Preheat the oven to 400°F. Spread the salt, pepper, and garlic on the filet mignon. Place in a roasting pan with red wine and beef broth and roast for 10 minutes. Reduce heat to 350°F and add the vegetables. Baste every 5 minutes.

2. Roast the filet mignon for another 20 minutes for medium-rare. Continue basting, turning the vegetables every 8–10 minutes.

3. Let the meat rest. Serve sliced and surrounded with potatoes, vegetables, and Mustard Cream Sauce (Hot).

PER SERVING (SAUCE NOT INCLUDED): Calories: 416 | GI: Low | Carbohydrates: 8g | Protein: 46g | Fat: 15g

CHAPTER 12

Pork, Lamb, and Veal Dishes

Scalloped Potato and Sausage Casserole with Greens

This recipe is another creative way to get your family to eat vegetables. Among the bits of sausage, your family will hardly notice them. The spices in the sausage will perfume the potatoes and veggies.

INGREDIENTS | SERVES 4

1 teaspoon vegetable oil

8 ounces lean pork breakfast sausage, crumbled

1 yellow onion, sliced

1 small zucchini, ends removed, diced

1 10-ounce package chopped frozen spinach, thawed and squeezed of moisture

¼ teaspoon nutmeg

Salt and pepper, to taste

Nonstick spray, as needed

2 Idaho or other russet potatoes, peeled and thinly sliced

¼ cup Parmesan cheese, grated

⅔ cup 2% milk

½ cup bread crumbs

1. Heat the oil in a large frying pan and sauté the sausage, onion, and zucchini. Stir to break up the sausage and mix well.

2. Stir in the spinach, nutmeg, salt, and pepper. Set aside.

3. Prepare a 9" pie plate with nonstick spray. Cover the bottom with half the sliced potatoes, add the sausage filling, and cover the top with the rest of the potatoes. Sprinkle with cheese and add milk.

4. Cover the top with bread crumbs; press down to moisten with milk. Bake for 50 minutes at 325°F, or until the potatoes are soft.

> **TIP:** *Substitute nonfat milk for 2% milk and replace sausage with vegetarian sausage.*

PER SERVING: Calories: 277 | GI: Moderate | Carbohydrates: 50g | Protein: 13g | Fat: 5g

Lamb Shanks with White Beans and Carrots

*This is a French bistro and comfort meal that most
people find delicious on a cool evening.*

INGREDIENTS | SERVES 4

4 lamb shanks, well trimmed

Salt and pepper, to taste

1 tablespoon olive oil

1 large yellow onion, chopped

4 garlic cloves, minced

1 carrot, peeled and cut into chunks

2 tablespoons tomato paste

1 cup dry red wine

1 cup chicken broth

2 bay leaves

¼ cup parsley, chopped

2 13-ounce cans white beans, drained
and rinsed

1. Sprinkle the lamb shanks with salt and pepper; brown in the olive oil, adding onion, garlic, and carrot. Cook for 5 minutes. Stir in tomato paste, red wine, chicken broth, bay leaves, and parsley.

2. Cover the pot and simmer for 1 hour. Add white beans and simmer for another 30 minutes. Remove bay leaves before serving.

PER SERVING: Calories: 417 | GI: Very low | Carbohydrates: 44g | Protein: 31g | Fat: 12g

Not Crazy about Lamb?

When people don't like lamb, it's usually the fat, not the lamb, they dislike. When you prepare roast lamb, stew, or shanks, be sure to remove all of the fat.

Country-Style Pork Ribs

*These big, meaty ribs are delicious when properly cooked. If you don't have a smoker,
add some wood chips to your grill, and if you don't have a grill, use a couple of drops of liquid smoke.
Serve with German-Style Potato Salad (see Chapter 15) and Old-Town Cole Slaw (see Chapter 15).*

INGREDIENTS | SERVES 4

2½ pounds country-style pork ribs

Salt and pepper, to taste

Garlic powder, to taste

Cayenne pepper, to taste

1 cup water

1 teaspoon liquid smoke

2 tablespoons Worcestershire sauce

1 cup any good barbecue sauce

Liquid Smoke

Liquid smoke is a flavoring for food used to give a smoky, barbecued flavor without the wood chips. It is most often made out of hickory wood, which producers burn to capture and condense the smoke. They filter out impurities in the liquid and bottle the rest.

1. Sprinkle the ribs with salt and pepper, garlic powder, and cayenne pepper. Rub the spices into the meat and bone on both sides. Place them in a turkey roasting pan with the water and liquid smoke on the bottom. Sprinkle with Worcestershire sauce.

2. Set the oven at 225°F. Cover the ribs tightly with aluminum foil. Roast them for 4–5 hours. They should be "falling off the bone" tender.

3. Remove foil and brush the ribs with barbecue sauce. Bake for another 15–20 minutes or until dark brown.

PER SERVING: Calories: 186 | GI: Low | Carbohydrates: 25g | Protein: 5g | Fat: 7g

Roast Leg of Veal

It may take a trip to the Internet to find a veal roast; however, if you can get a young one, it's fabulous. A crisp salad, asparagus, or broccoli make excellent accompaniments.

INGREDIENTS | SERVES 8

1 5-pound veal leg roast, shank half of the leg, bone in

1 tablespoon prepared mustard, Dijon-style

2 tablespoons all-purpose flour

1 tablespoon butter, at room temperature

1 teaspoon dried sage, crumbled

2 teaspoons dried rosemary, crumbled

Salt and freshly ground black pepper, to taste

1 cup chicken broth

½ cup dry white wine

1. Make sure the veal is well trimmed and has no skin on it. Set oven at 400°F. Make a paste of the mustard, flour, butter, herbs, salt, and pepper. Coat the veal with the mustard mixture.

2. Place veal in a roasting pan and place in the hot, preheated oven. Roast for 15 minutes. Turn down heat and baste with ¼ cup chicken broth and ¼ cup wine for 15 minutes.

3. Reduce heat to 325°F. Continue to roast and baste the meat with remaining broth and wine for another 45 minutes, or until the internal temperature reaches 150°F.

4. Let the meat rest on a platter for 15 minutes before carving. Serve with pan juices; if dry, add ½ cup boiling water to pan and whisk.

TIP: *Replace butter with olive oil or heart-healthy margarine.*

PER SERVING: Calories: 174 | GI: Zero | Carbohydrates: 1g | Protein: 22g | Fat: 7g

Grilled Rib Lamb Chops with Garlic and Citrus

Young lamb is a great party dish and is perfect when cooked medium-rare.

INGREDIENTS | SERVES 2

2 teaspoons olive oil

½ lemon, juice and zest

1 tablespoon grapefruit juice

1–2 cloves garlic, minced

1 teaspoon dried rosemary, or 1 tablespoon fresh

Salt and pepper, to taste

8 baby rib lamb chops, about ½" each, well trimmed

2 tablespoons white vermouth, for basting

1. Using a mortar and pestle, mash the olive oil, lemon juice and zest, grapefruit juice, garlic, rosemary, salt, and pepper.

2. Make sure all fat is removed from the lamb chops. Coat lamb chops with the garlic mixture and let rest in the refrigerator for 1 hour.

3. Heat grill to high. Place chops over high flame until seared on one side. Baste with vermouth and turn after 3 minutes. Baste again and reduce heat. Cover the grill and let chops roast for 8 minutes.

PER SERVING: Calories: 513 | GI: Zero | Carbohydrates: 0g | Protein: 68g | Fat: 24g

Mini Spinach Casserole with Ricotta Cheese, Brown Rice, and Ham

This is a delicious way to keep your GI low while getting nutrients.

INGREDIENTS | SERVES 2

2 cups fresh baby spinach

½ cup low-fat ricotta cheese

Salt and pepper, to taste

1 cup brown rice, cooked

¼ cup Italian Dressing (see Chapter 6)

1 ounce Virginia ham, chopped

Purée the spinach and ricotta in the blender. Preheat oven to 300°F. Mix all ingredients together in a 9" pie pan and bake for 20 minutes.

PER SERVING: Calories: 342 | GI: Low | Carbohydrates: 32g | Protein: 16g | Fat: 19g

Pork Tenderloin with Caraway Sauerkraut

Caraway is a popular flavor in Scandinavian and eastern European cooking.
It is excellent with veal and pork. Tenderloin of pork is lean, moist, and delicious.
It is very low in calories and a real treat with the sauerkraut.

INGREDIENTS | SERVES 2

1 teaspoon olive oil
8 ounces pork tenderloin
Salt and pepper, to taste
1 teaspoon Wondra flour
2 medium red onions, chopped
¼ cup low-salt chicken broth
8 ounces sauerkraut, drained
1 teaspoon caraway seeds

1. Heat the oil in a frying pan over medium heat. Sprinkle the pork tenderloin with salt, pepper, and flour. Sauté the pork over medium heat for 4 minutes; turn the pork and add onions.

2. Continue to sauté until the pork is lightly browned on both sides and the onions have softened slightly.

3. Add the chicken broth, sauerkraut, and caraway seeds. Cover and simmer for 25 minutes. Pork should be pink.

PER SERVING: Calories: 309 | GI: Zero | Carbohydrates: 4g | Protein: 36g | Fat: 15g

Pork-Stuffed Wontons over Napa Cabbage

This recipe combines Eastern and Western flavors in a low GI, high-energy meal.

INGREDIENTS | SERVES 4

½ cup sweet onion, finely chopped

2 cloves garlic, minced

2 ounces peanut oil

½ pound ground pork

1 ounce soy sauce

2 ounces raisins

1 ounce pine nuts, toasted

Salt and pepper, to taste

24 wonton wrappers

Nonstick spray, as needed

Double recipe Napa Cabbage with Asian Sauce (see Chapter 15)

Wrap It Up

Thin wonton wrappers are available at many supermarkets and all Asian markets. You can use them to make fast and easy ravioli, dumplings, or wonton soup, or you can fry the wrappers alone and top with grilled or stir-fried veggies and steak.

1. Make the stuffing by sautéing onion and garlic in the peanut oil. When softened, mix in pork, stirring to break up lumps.

2. Mix in the soy sauce, raisins, pine nuts, salt, and pepper.

3. Divide the pork stuffing among wonton wrappers and moisten edges with a bit of water before folding into triangles. At this point, wontons can be stored in refrigerator for a day or frozen for a month.

4. Steam wontons in a steamer prepared with nonstick spray for 10 minutes.

5. Serve over cabbage.

PER SERVING: Calories: 635 | GI: Very low | Carbohydrates: 55g | Protein: 30g | Fat: 33g

Veal Piquant with Ratatouille

Using a vegetable stew as a base for meats keeps the GI of your meal low and makes for a lovely presentation.

INGREDIENTS | SERVES 2

½ pound veal, thinly sliced and pounded

Salt and pepper, to taste

1 tablespoon flour

1 tablespoon olive oil

1 recipe Ratatouille with White Beans (see Chapter 9)

Juice of ½ lemon

1 teaspoon capers

1 tablespoon fresh rosemary, chopped

1 tablespoon fresh parsley, chopped

½ cup chicken broth

Additions and Substitutions

To add substance to this dish, you can use a mound of polenta as a base. You can also substitute chicken breasts instead of veal.

1. Dress the veal with salt, pepper, and a dusting of flour. Heat the olive oil at medium-high. Sauté veal very quickly, about 2 minutes per side. Place on a heated serving platter.

2. Prepare the Ratatouille with White Beans. Using the pan in which the veal was cooked, add the lemon juice, capers, and herbs.

3. Stir in the chicken broth. Reduce over medium heat. Just before serving, return the veal to the pan and turn to coat with sauce. Pour the rest of the sauce over the veal and serve.

PER SERVING (NOT INCLUDING RATATOUILLE): Calories: 267 | GI: Very low | Carbohydrates: 5g | Protein: 29g | Fat: 14g

Pan-Fried Pork Chops with Apple

Apple and rosemary pair perfectly with pork chops.

INGREDIENTS | SERVES 4

4 boneless pork loin chops

2 teaspoons olive oil

2 tablespoons fresh rosemary, chopped

¼ teaspoon salt

½ teaspoon fresh ground pepper

1 medium Granny Smith apple, cored and quartered

¼ cup golden raisins

¾ cup red wine

Nonstick spray, as needed

1. Rub pork chops lightly with 1 teaspoon olive oil. Combine rosemary, salt, and pepper, and rub evenly on both sides of pork chops.

2. In a hot skillet, add remaining oil and cook apple and raisins over medium heat, stirring, for 4 minutes.

3. Add half the wine, continuously stirring, until liquid evaporates. Add remaining wine and cook on medium-low heat for 15 minutes.

4. In a pan covered with cooking spray over medium heat, cook pork chops for 6 minutes on each side. Serve chops with apple mixture.

PER SERVING: Calories: 273 | GI: Low | Carbohydrates: 15g | Protein: 35g | Fat: 6g

Country Ham

A country ham is a beautiful thing! Depending on where they come from, country hams are smoked or salt cured. Both are improved by soaking.

INGREDIENTS | SERVES 20

10-pound country ham, bone in
Water, to cover
10 bay leaves
1 pound brown sugar, plus ½ cup
20 whole cloves, bruised
25 peppercorns, bruised
10 coriander seeds, bruised
2 tablespoons dark mustard
½ teaspoon powdered cloves
1½ cups apple cider

1. Prepare the ham by removing skin and most of the fat, leaving ¼" of fat.

2. Place ham in large container and add water to cover. Add bay leaves, 1 pound brown sugar, cloves, peppercorns, and coriander seeds; soak for 30 hours.

3. Preheat the oven to 300°F. Pat the ham dry and place in a roasting pan. Mix the rest of the brown sugar with the mustard and powdered cloves; spread on the ham.

4. Bake for 3½ hours, basting with the apple cider. You can degrease the pan juices and use the apple cider as a sauce; otherwise, serve with applesauce.

PER SERVING (NOT INCLUDING APPLE CIDER): Calories: 403 | GI: Low | Carbohydrates: 0g | Protein: 51g | Fat: 21g

Broiled Lamb Chops with Mint Chimichurri Sauce

Forget mint jelly. Here, chimichurri, an Argentinian herb sauce, is front and center.

INGREDIENTS | SERVES 4

2 cloves garlic
1 tablespoon olive oil
1 teaspoon salt
1 teaspoon black pepper
4 4-ounce lamb chops
1 recipe Mint Chimichurri Sauce (see Chapter 14)

1. Mash garlic cloves. Mix with olive oil to form a paste. Add salt and pepper to the paste. Spread garlic paste evenly on the 4 chops.

2. Broil lamb chops until browned but slightly pink inside, about 4–5 minutes per side.

3. Serve with Mint Chimichurri Sauce.

PER SERVING: Calories: 178 | GI: Very low | Carbohydrates: 0g | Protein: 24g | Fat: 8g

Grilled Lamb Chops with Garlic, Rosemary, and Thyme

These succulent lamb chops are inspired by typical flavors of Greek cuisine.

INGREDIENTS | SERVES 2

2 cloves garlic
½ teaspoon salt
1 teaspoon fresh rosemary, chopped
1 teaspoon fresh thyme, chopped
1 tablespoon olive oil
1 teaspoon lemon zest, minced
Pepper, to taste
4 1¼"-thick lamb chops

1. Mash garlic cloves into a paste. Add salt.

2. In a bowl, stir together garlic paste, rosemary, thyme, oil, and lemon zest, and add pepper to taste. Rub the herb-garlic paste onto the lamb chops and set them aside to marinate for 15 minutes.

3. Grill lamb chops for 4–5 minutes on each side for medium-rare doneness.

PER SERVING: Calories: 287 | GI: Very low | Carbohydrates: 1g | Protein: 35g | Fat: 15g

Curried Lamb

Shoulder lamb chops work best for this inexpensive dish. Remember that when buying meat on the bone for a recipe that you have to allow for the weight of the bones. The bones add a great deal of flavor to stews and soups, even though you have to take them out later.

INGREDIENTS | SERVES 4

2 tablespoons canola oil

2 pounds shoulder lamb chops, bone in, trimmed of fat

4 white onions, chopped

4 cloves garlic, chopped

2 serrano or Scotch bonnet chilies, cored, seeded, and chopped

1" gingerroot, peeled and minced

2 carrots, peeled and chopped

1 stalk celery with leaves, chopped

2 fresh tomatoes, chopped

1 roasted red pepper, chopped

1 cup chicken broth

2 tablespoons curry powder

½ cup dry white wine

Salt and pepper, to taste

1. Heat the canola oil over medium flame in a large pot. Brown the lamb and then add the rest of the vegetables.

2. Stir in the chicken broth. Mix the curry powder with the white wine to dissolve it and stir into the pot. Season with salt and pepper.

3. Cover the pot and reduce heat to a simmer. Cook over very low heat for 3 hours. Cool and remove the bones and any fat that has come to the top of the stew.

4. Reheat just before serving.

PER SERVING: Calories: 420 | GI: Zero | Carbohydrates: 22g | Protein: 37g | Fat: 19g

Hawaiian Fresh Ham, Roasted with Pineapple and Rum

Fresh ham is basically leg of pork.
It is a tender white meat and a great fall or winter dish.

INGREDIENTS | SERVES 10

2 cups pineapple juice

1 cup rum

¼ cup brown sugar, or to taste

½ teaspoon cloves, ground

Salt and hot red pepper sauce, to taste

6 pounds fresh ham, some fat (about ¼")

1 fresh pineapple, peeled and cut into chunks

1. Preheat oven to 350°F. Reduce the pineapple juice to 1 cup over high heat. Add rum, brown sugar, cloves, salt, and red pepper sauce.

2. Score the fat left on the ham with a sharp knife and place ham in a roasting pan. Baste with pineapple syrup. Roast and baste for 3 hours, basting often. If the bottom of the pan starts to burn, add water.

3. Surround with the fresh pineapple chunks in the last hour of cooking. If the ham gets too brown, tent with aluminum foil.

4. Serve with the pan drippings on the side and caramelized pineapple chunks, also on the side.

PER SERVING: Calories: 608 | GI: Low | Carbohydrates: 27g | Protein: 28g | Fat: 37g

Pork Chops with Balsamic Glaze

Shallots, balsamic vinegar, and agave nectar add a balanced touch of sweetness to this savory dish.

INGREDIENTS | SERVES 4

4 5-ounce center-cut pork chops
1 teaspoon salt
Fresh ground pepper, to taste
2 tablespoons olive oil
6 large shallots, peeled and quartered
½ cup balsamic vinegar
2 teaspoons agave nectar

1. Wash and pat dry the pork chops. Season pork with ½ teaspoon salt and pepper.

2. Heat oil in a large pan over medium-high heat. Cook pork and shallots in pan. Turn pork over once to cook about 3 minutes on each side, and stir shallots occasionally until tender. Transfer pork to a plate, cover, and set aside.

3. Add vinegar, agave nectar, ½ teaspoon salt, and a pinch of pepper to shallots in the pan. Cook until liquid begins to thicken, about 1–2 minutes.

4. Turn heat down to medium-low; return pork back to the pan and coat well with sauce. Cook for 3–4 minutes; a thermometer inserted into pork should read 150°F.

5. Remove pork from the pan, turn heat up, and allow remaining sauce to thicken. Pour sauce over pork chops before serving.

PER SERVING: Calories: 284 | GI: Low | Carbohydrates: 11g | Protein: 25g | Fat: 11g

Veal Steaks

*Veal, known for its tender texture and unique flavor,
has been a common ingredient in French and Italian cooking since ancient times.*

INGREDIENTS | SERVES 4

Nonstick cooking spray, as needed

2 teaspoons olive oil

2 tablespoons whole-wheat flour

¼ teaspoon white pepper

4 boneless veal steaks

2 large shallots, minced

½ cup low-sodium beef broth

½ cup red cooking wine

2 teaspoons Dijon mustard

2 tablespoons capers

½ cup low-fat sour cream

1. Coat a large pan with nonstick cooking spray and add oil. Combine flour and pepper; dredge veal steaks through flour-pepper mixture. Place pan over medium-high heat and, when hot, add veal and shallots. Cook until veal is browned on both sides, about 3–4 minutes per side.

2. Drain excess oil from the pan. Mix beef broth, wine, mustard, and capers and pour over veal. Turn heat up to high, bring to a boil, cover, and reduce heat to a simmer for 20–25 minutes. Transfer veal steaks to a plate, cover, and set aside.

3. Bring remaining broth in the pan to a boil; cook, uncovered, over medium heat until broth is reduced in half. Remove pan from heat, add sour cream, and mix well until blended. Serve sauce with veal steaks.

PER SERVING: Calories: 235 | GI: Low | Carbohydrates: 6g | Protein: 25g | Fat: 10g

CHAPTER 13

Fish and Seafood

Raw Oysters on the Half Shell with Mignonette Sauce

This is a wonderful holiday appetizer. You can make the mignonette sauce in advance.
Oysters should be served the day they are opened. Tell your fishmonger
not to rinse off the liquor (natural juice). The oyster liquor is full of great flavor!

INGREDIENTS | SERVES 2

2 shallots, minced
1 tablespoon lemon juice
1 tablespoon Italian parsley, chopped
Salt and pepper, to taste
½ cup extra-virgin olive oil
12 raw oysters, on the half shell, resting on a bed of ice

Place the shallots, lemon juice, parsley, salt, and pepper in the blender. On low speed, slowly add the olive oil. Spoon over the oysters.

PER SERVING: Calories: 155 | GI: Zero | Carbohydrates: 7g | Protein: 7g | Fat: 11g

Baked Oysters with Shrimp Stuffing

This recipe is perfect for those who would rather eat their oysters cooked.
Always taste the liquor for saltiness. Some oysters are very salty; some are not.
This is an easy recipe for a romantic dinner, or you can just add to it for a party.

INGREDIENTS | SERVES 2

1 teaspoon butter
2 shallots, chopped
2 slices bacon, fried and crumbled
1 tablespoon lemon juice
2 slices stale white bread, crumbled
8 raw oysters, on the half shell, liquor reserved
4 medium shrimp, raw, peeled, deveined, and chopped
Salt, if necessary
Plenty of freshly ground pepper

1. Set oven at 425°F. Melt the butter; add shallots and sauté for 5 minutes on medium heat. Add the crumbled bacon and lemon juice.

2. Stir in the bread crumbs and mix in the oyster liquor. Add shrimp, salt to taste, and grind on pepper.

3. Divide the bread and shrimp mixture among the oysters. Bake for 12–15 minutes, or until the oysters are bubbling and the topping is well browned.

TIP: *Substitute vegetarian "bacon" for regular bacon and replace butter with olive oil.*

PER SERVING: Calories: 222 | GI: Low | Carbohydrates: 20g | Protein: 16g | Fat: 10g

Regional Oysters

Depending on where they come from, oysters can have different flavors. Some oysters are extremely sweet and light in flavor. Some Pacific Coast oysters taste metallic, and oysters from certain estuaries have a distinctly swampy flavor. Oysters from Long Island Sound are exported to Japan and France and are very sweet tasting.

Grilled Tuna Steak with Vegetables and Pine Nuts

Grilled tuna is a favorite of dieters. The Asian vegetables in this recipe add some carbohydrates necessary for good health.

INGREDIENTS | SERVES 2

1 cup napa cabbage, shredded

½ cup pea pods, coarsely chopped

½ cup carrots, shredded

3 tablespoons tomato sauce

¼ cup pine nuts, toasted

2 tuna steaks, ¼ pound each

1 teaspoon sesame oil

1 teaspoon lime juice

Salt and pepper, to taste

1. Poach the vegetables in the tomato sauce for 8 minutes or until crisp-tender. Add the pine nuts and set aside.

2. Set grill on medium-high. Spread the tuna with sesame oil, lime juice, salt, and pepper. Grill for 4 minutes per side for medium.

3. Serve with tomato-poached vegetables.

PER SERVING: Calories: 277 | GI: Zero | Carbohydrates: 25g | Protein: 18g | Fat: 13g

Salmon and Broccoli Stir-Fry

This is a quick and easy supper, in addition to being good for you.
You can blanch the broccoli in advance.

INGREDIENTS | SERVES 2

½ pound broccoli florets

½ pound salmon fillet, skin removed

1 tablespoon canola oil

1 teaspoon Asian sesame oil

1 teaspoon gingerroot, minced

2 slices pickled ginger, chopped

1 clove garlic, minced

1 teaspoon hoisin sauce

Optional: 1 cup brown rice

Garnish of 5 scallions, chopped

1. Blanch the broccoli in boiling water for 5 minutes; drain.

2. Toss the broccoli and salmon over medium-high heat with the canola oil and sesame oil. Cook, stirring for 3–4 minutes.

3. Add the gingerroot, pickled ginger, garlic, and hoisin sauce and serve over rice, garnished with scallions.

PER SERVING: Calories: 273 | GI: Zero | Carbohydrates: 7g | Protein: 25g | Fat: 6g

Food Safety

When preparing a dish that lists fish, seafood, or poultry as one of the ingredients, be sure to keep the fish, seafood, or chicken ice-cold during preparation to ensure food safety. If you will be doing a lot of handling or if the food will be on the counter for a long time, keep a bowl with ice nearby to place the ingredients in while you are tending to other steps of the recipe.

Roast Stuffed Striped Bass

This is very festive, and you can serve a mob by multiplying the recipe.

INGREDIENTS | SERVES 2

2 slices whole-grain bread, toasted

1 stalk celery, finely chopped

¼ cup parsley, chopped

2 tablespoons unsalted butter, melted

½ cup canned water chestnuts

1 tablespoon lemon juice

Salt and pepper, to taste

¾-pound fillet striped bass, skin on

1. Place everything but the striped bass in the food processor or blender. Pulse until well crumbled.

2. Set oven on 350°F. Place striped bass on a baking sheet. Spread stuffing on fish.

3. Bake the fish for 12–15 minutes, or until the stuffing is well browned.

TIP: *Substitute olive oil for butter.*

PER SERVING: Calories: 395 | GI: Low | Carbohydrates: 22g | Protein: 36g | Fat: 19g

Stripers

Striped bass are native to a large portion of the East Coast and range as far south as northern Florida. The fish has lean, white meat and a mild flavor, and it is especially tasty when stuffed with vegetables and bread crumbs or grilled.

Baked Fillet of Sole with Shrimp Sauce and Artichokes

The varieties of sole are daunting. There's gray, lemon, Dover, and more.
When you are buying sole, make sure that it smells like fresh milk. Get whatever is cheapest—
it will taste pretty much the same from lemon to gray to Dover. All taste delicious when fresh!

INGREDIENTS | SERVES 2

5 medium shrimp, cooked

1 shallot, chopped

¼ cup low-fat mayonnaise

¼ teaspoon dill, dried

2 tablespoons orange juice

1 9-ounce package frozen artichoke hearts

2 6-ounce sole fillets

Nonstick spray, as needed

Salt and pepper, to taste

4 tablespoons fine dry bread crumbs

Artichokes

Artichokes are thistle-like plants, and the part we eat is actually the immature flower head. There are many varieties, but the type commonly available in the United States (usually in markets November through May) are globe artichokes. The soft heart or center of the artichoke can be eaten raw or cooked sprinkled with olive oil, salt, and pepper.

1. Preheat oven to 375°F. Pulse the shrimp, shallot, mayonnaise, dill, and orange juice in the blender. Set the sauce aside.

2. Cook the frozen artichokes to package directions. Place sole on a baking sheet prepared with nonstick spray. Sprinkle the fillets with salt and pepper. Arrange the artichokes around the sole. Spoon sauce over all. Sprinkle with bread crumbs.

3. Bake for 15 minutes, or until the sole is hot and bubbling and the artichokes are crisply browned on top.

PER SERVING: Calories: 368 | GI: Very low | Carbohydrates: 20g | Protein: 43g | Fat: 13g

Shrimp and Vegetables over Napa Cabbage

This recipe takes little time to prepare and is packed with both flavor and energy-boosting ingredients.

INGREDIENTS | SERVES 2

1 tablespoon peanut oil

1 clove garlic, minced

1 teaspoon sesame seeds

1 carrot, shredded

½ large zucchini, shredded

½ cup jicama, peeled and finely chopped

¼ cup dry white wine

1 tablespoon lemon juice

1 ounce dry sherry

½ pound raw shrimp, peeled and deveined

1 recipe Napa Cabbage with Asian Sauce (see Chapter 15)

1. In a large frying pan over medium heat, add the peanut oil, garlic, and sesame seeds and sauté, stirring for 5 minutes. Add the vegetables and mix. Pour in the wine and lemon juice. Simmer to burn off alcohol; cover.

2. When the vegetables are crisp-tender, add the sherry and shrimp. Stir and cook until the shrimp turn pink. Serve with Napa Cabbage with Asian Sauce.

PER SERVING: Calories: 213 | GI: Very low | Carbohydrates: 15g | Protein: 5g | Fat: 11g

Corn-Crusted Salmon with Parsley and Radish Topping

*This is a festive way to prepare salmon, and it's very pretty
with the colorful green parsley and red radishes.*

INGREDIENTS | SERVES 2

4 radishes, thinly sliced

½ cup parsley, Italian flat-leaf, minced

1 tablespoon olive oil

2 tablespoons red wine vinegar

½ teaspoon celery salt

2 salmon fillets, about 6 ounces each

1 tablespoon lemon juice

¼ cup cornmeal

¼ cup 2% milk

½ teaspoon dill, dried

3 tablespoons olive oil

Red pepper flakes, to taste

Nonstick spray, as needed

1. Mix the radishes, parsley, olive oil, vinegar, and celery salt. Set aside.

2. Make sure the salmon has no pin bones; sprinkle with lemon juice. Mix together the cornmeal, milk, dill, olive oil, and red pepper flakes. Spread on the salmon and rest it in the refrigerator for ½ hour.

3. Set oven at 350°F. Prepare a baking dish or metal sheet with nonstick spray. Place salmon on the baking dish or sheet.

4. Bake the salmon for 20 minutes, or until the topping is brown and the salmon flakes. Serve with radish-parsley topping.

TIP: *Substitute nonfat milk for 2% milk in the topping for the salmon in this recipe.*

PER SERVING: Calories: 371 | GI: Very low | Carbohydrates: 10g | Protein: 36g | Fat: 21g

Pistachio-Crusted Halibut

A nut crust on fish is a healthier alternative to the typical bread-crumb crust and packs just as much of a crunch.

INGREDIENTS | SERVES 2

2 6-ounce skinless halibut fillets
½ cup low-fat milk
¼ cup shelled pistachios
1½ tablespoons cornmeal
1 teaspoon garlic powder
⅛ teaspoon cayenne pepper
¼ teaspoon salt
Freshly ground white pepper, to taste
2 tablespoons olive oil

Fun Facts

Did you know that during harvesting season, pistachio trees are shaken to remove the nuts from the branches? Pistachios must be shelled before eaten, one by one, and therefore the body is fooled into thinking more nuts have been consumed. This concept of tricking the mind into telling the body to eat less is sometimes called the Pistachio Principle.

1. Place fillets in a glass baking dish. Pour milk over top, cover, and chill for 30 minutes.

2. Toast pistachios lightly and chop finely with a chef's knife. Mix together pistachios, cornmeal, garlic powder, and cayenne pepper in a bowl.

3. Remove fish from the milk, season with salt and white pepper, then dredge in pistachio mixture. Place fillets on a clean plate.

4. Heat oil in a large pan over medium-high heat. Once oil is hot, sauté fillets 3–4 minutes per side, until lightly browned on the outside and cooked through in the center.

PER SERVING: Calories: 484 | GI: Low | Carbohydrates: 13g | Protein: 49g | Fat: 26g

Garlic Shrimp with Bok Choy

Bok choy is a Chinese cabbage that is staggeringly simple to prepare and is rich in many important nutrients including vitamin A, vitamin C, and folate.

INGREDIENTS | SERVES 2

1 tablespoon sesame oil
3 cloves garlic, chopped
1 tablespoon fresh ginger, grated
1 pound bok choy cabbage
1 cup broccoli florets
1 pound shrimp, peeled and deveined
¼ cup low-sodium soy sauce

1. Heat oil in a pan or wok over medium-high heat. Add garlic and ginger, stir, and cook for 30 seconds.

2. Turn heat up to high. Add bok choy and broccoli and stir-fry for 2–3 minutes. Add shrimp and continue stirring.

3. Add soy sauce and cook until shrimp are pink and completely done.

PER SERVING: Calories: 175 | GI: Low | Carbohydrates: 6g | Protein: 25g | Fat: 6g

Cod with Tomatoes and Garlic

Cooked tomatoes are an excellent source of lycopene, which possesses antioxidant properties important for eye health.

INGREDIENTS | SERVES 6

2 pounds cod fillet
2 tablespoons olive oil, divided
4 teaspoons salt, divided
1 teaspoon black pepper, divided
2 large tomatoes, sliced ¼" thick
2 medium onions, sliced
3 cloves garlic, minced
2 tablespoons capers
1 tablespoon Italian seasoning

1. Preheat oven to 400°F.

2. Rinse cod and pat dry. Season the fish with 1 tablespoon olive oil, 3 teaspoons salt, and ½ teaspoon black pepper. Place in a glass baking dish.

3. In a medium bowl, combine tomatoes, onions, garlic, capers, Italian seasoning, 1 tablespoon olive oil, 1 teaspoon salt, and ½ teaspoon black pepper.

4. Place tomato and garlic mixture evenly over top of the cod. Place dish in the oven and bake 20 minutes.

PER SERVING: Calories: 204 | GI: Very low | Carbohydrates: 6g | Protein: 31g | Fat: 6g

Lemon-Garlic Shrimp and Vegetables

The shrimp will sing in this light stir-fry with hints of sweet and sour flavors.

INGREDIENTS | SERVES 2

2 tablespoons low-sodium soy sauce

1 teaspoon lemon zest

1½ tablespoons lemon juice

½ teaspoon agave nectar

½ cup water

Black pepper, to taste

Nonstick spray, as needed

1 celery stalk, sliced

1 cup red cabbage, shredded

½ red bell pepper, thinly sliced

3 cloves garlic, chopped

½ cup bean sprouts

1 teaspoon sesame oil

½ pound raw shrimp, peeled and deveined

1. Mix soy sauce, lemon zest, lemon juice, agave nectar, water, and pepper in a small bowl; set aside.

2. Spray a large pan with nonstick cooking spray. Place pan over medium heat.

3. Add celery and cabbage to the pan; sauté for 1 minute. Add bell pepper, garlic, and bean sprouts, and sauté until all vegetables are crisp-tender. Transfer vegetable to a plate and cover.

4. Add oil to the pan, and once oil is hot, place shrimp in the hot pan and cook until opaque. Return vegetables to the pan with the cooked shrimp.

5. Pour soy sauce mixture over the shrimp and vegetables and cook for 3–4 minutes, until sauce has reduced.

PER SERVING: Calories: 190 | GI: Low | Carbohydrates: 11g | Protein: 26g | Fat: 4g

Mahi Mahi Tacos with Avocado and Fresh Cabbage

These California-style tacos can be prepared with any meaty, mild fish or shrimp.

INGREDIENTS | MAKES 4 TACOS

1 pound mahi mahi

Salt and pepper, to taste

1 teaspoon olive oil

1 avocado

4 corn tortillas

2 cups cabbage, shredded

2 limes, quartered

Salsa Verde

Fish tacos taste great with a citrusy salsa to brighten them up. Try these fish tacos accompanied by Salsa Verde (see Chapter 14). You'll love this combination!

1. Season fish with salt and pepper. Heat oil in a large pan over medium heat. Once the oil is hot, sauté fish for about 3–4 minutes on each side. Slice or flake fish into 1-ounce pieces

2. Slice avocado in half. Remove seed and, using a spoon, remove the flesh from the skin. Slice the avocado halves into ½"-thick slices.

3. In a small pan, warm corn tortillas; cook for about 1 minute on each side.

4. Place one-fourth of mahi mahi on each tortilla; top with avocado and cabbage. Serve with lime wedges.

PER SERVING: Calories: 251 | GI: Low | Carbohydrates: 21g | Protein: 25g | Fat: 9g

Planked Salmon with Dill Sauce

This is a very festive and delicious way to prepare salmon.
The use of a cedar plank and juniper berries are reminiscent of Native American cooking.

INGREDIENTS | SERVES 10

1 cedar plank

Water, as needed

Grapeseed oil, as needed

3½ pounds salmon fillet, checked for bones

Juice of 1 lemon

8 juniper berries

Salt and pepper, to taste

1 lemon, thinly sliced

1 cup mayonnaise

¼ cup fresh dill weed, chopped

1 teaspoon horseradish

Fish Bones

The larger the fish, the more likely you will find bones in a fillet. Before cooking, hold a clean pair of pliers and run the finger of your other hand down the fillet, against the grain. Whenever you feel a bone, press down close to it. It will pop up, and you can then pull it out with the pliers.

1. Soak the plank in water. When thoroughly soaked, lightly oil the side on which the salmon will lay. Set the salmon on the plank. Sprinkle with lemon juice and press the juniper berries into the flesh at intervals. Add salt, pepper, and lemon slices.

2. Place the plank over indirect heat on a hot grill and close lid. Roast for about 15–20 minutes or until the salmon begins to flake.

3. Mix the rest of the ingredients together in a small bowl with more salt and pepper and serve with the fish.

TIP: *In this recipe, you can substitute low-fat mayonnaise for regular mayonnaise.*

PER SERVING: Calories: 388 | GI: Zero | Carbohydrates: 2g | Protein: 32g | Fat: 28g

Smoked Salmon, Eggs, and Cheese Puffed Casserole

This is an excellent brunch dish. Serve with a salad on the side and feast!

INGREDIENTS | SERVES 2

4 eggs, separated

2 slices whole-grain bread

4 ounces cream cheese, at room temperature

½ cup white onion, chopped

Pepper, to taste

¼ cup 2% milk

Nonstick spray, as needed

⅛ pound smoked salmon

Omega-3 Fatty Acids

Salmon is an excellent source of omega-3 fatty acids, which can improve heart function and lower blood pressure. You can get omega-3 fatty acids from most cold-water fish, such as albacore tuna, salmon, and trout, which tend to have more of these good fats than other fish.

1. Preheat the oven to 400°F. Beat the egg whites until stiff and set aside. Cut bread into quarters.

2. Place the egg yolks, cream cheese, onion, pepper, bread, and milk in the food processor or blender and purée until smooth and creamy.

3. Prepare a 1-quart soufflé dish with nonstick spray; place bread in the bottom of the dish. In a bowl, fold the beaten egg whites into the cheese mixture and gently mix in the salmon. Pour into the dish.

4. Bake for 30 minutes or until puffed and golden.

TIP: *Substitute nonfat milk for 2% milk and replace sour cream with low-fat sour cream.*

PER SERVING: Calories: 478 | GI: Low | Carbohydrates: 20g | Protein: 27g | Fat: 33g

Asian Sesame-Crusted Scallops

Sea scallops can be grilled, broiled, or sautéed. Try to get really big scallops—called diver scallops. They are very sweet and velvety in texture. These are delicious as an appetizer for 4 or as a main course for 2.

INGREDIENTS | SERVES 2

2 cups napa cabbage, shredded

1 large ripe tomato, sliced

2 ounces soy sauce

1 ounce sesame oil

Juice of ½ lime

1" fresh gingerroot, peeled and minced

½ pound diver scallops, each weighing 1+ ounces (3–4 per person)

1 egg, beaten

½ cup sesame seeds

2 tablespoons peanut oil

Salt and pepper, to taste

1. Make beds on 2 serving plates with the cabbage and the tomatoes. In a small bowl, mix together the soy sauce, sesame oil, lime juice, and minced ginger to create sauce.

2. Rinse the scallops and pat them dry on paper towels. Dip scallops in beaten egg. Spread sesame seeds on waxed paper, and roll scallops in them to cover.

3. Heat the peanut oil in a nonstick frying pan. Sear the scallops over medium heat until browned on both sides and heated through. Do not overcook, or they will get tough. Arrange the scallops over the greens and tomatoes; add salt and pepper. Drizzle with the sauce.

PER SERVING: Calories: 272 | GI: Very low | Carbohydrates: 12g | Protein: 27g | Fat: 14g

Classic Parisian Mussels

This dish, from traditional French bistro cuisine, should be prepared using good quality white wine and fresh mussels.

INGREDIENTS | SERVES 4

2 tablespoons butter

½ white onion, minced

3 cloves garlic, minced

4 pounds mussels, cleaned

3 tablespoons flat-leaf parsley, chopped

1 bay leaf

5 whole black peppercorns

2 cups dry white wine

How to Clean Mussels

Soak the mussels in water for 20 minutes; discard dirty water. To remove the beard, grab it and sharply pull it toward the hinge side of the mussel. Before cooking, scrub with a brush under cold water. Throw away any mussels that are cracked or open.

1. Place a large stockpot over medium heat. Melt butter, then sauté onion and garlic until translucent.

2. Turn heat to high and add all additional ingredients to the pot. Bring contents to a boil, cover pot with lid, and cook until the mussels open, about 5 minutes.

3. Remove the pot from the heat. Transfer mussels to serving dish using a slotted spoon.

4. Using a ladle, spoon the broth from the pot over the mussels before serving. Be careful to leave any sand or sediment from the mussels behind in the bottom of the pot and remove bay leaves before serving.

PER SERVING: Calories: 436 | GI: Low | Carbohydrates: 18g | Protein: 33g | Fat: 13g

Jambalaya

An authentic Louisiana favorite full of flavor and spice.

INGREDIENTS | SERVES 6

1 tablespoon olive oil

2 chicken breasts, boneless and skinless, chopped

8 ounces andouille sausage, sliced

12 medium shrimp, peeled and deveined

½ medium onion, chopped

2 green bell peppers, chopped

2 stalks celery, diced

2 cloves garlic, minced

¼ teaspoon crushed red pepper

1 teaspoon chili powder

2 teaspoons dried oregano

Black pepper, to taste

6 ounces brown rice

2½ cans low-sodium chicken broth

1 can tomatoes, diced

1 cup water

Tabasco sauce, to taste

1. Pour oil into a large pot and place on medium-high heat. Sauté chicken and sausage until browned. Add shrimp; cook and stir until shrimp are opaque.

2. Add onion, bell pepper, celery, and garlic; season with crushed red pepper, chili powder, oregano, and black pepper. Cook until onion is tender.

3. Stir in rice, broth, tomatoes, and water. Bring to a boil and then reduce heat; simmer until rice is cooked. Stir in Tabasco before serving.

PER SERVING: Calories: 328 | GI: Moderate | Carbohydrates: 29g | Protein: 22g | Fat: 14g

Savory Fish Stew

This stew is fresh and easy with a whole lot of flavor.
The recipe calls for halibut, but just about any meaty white fish will do.

INGREDIENTS | SERVES 6

1 tablespoon olive oil
1 onion, finely chopped
½ cup dry white wine
3 large tomatoes, chopped
2 cups low-sodium chicken broth
8 ounces clam juice
3 cups fresh spinach
1 pound halibut fillets, cut into 1" pieces
White pepper, to taste
1 tablespoon fresh cilantro, chopped

1. Place a large pan over medium heat. Add oil to the pan and sauté onions for 2–3 minutes. Add wine to deglaze the pan. Scrape the pan to loosen small bits of onion.

2. Add tomatoes and cook for 3–4 minutes, then add broth and clam juice to the pan. Stir in spinach and allow to wilt while continuing to stir.

3. Season fish with pepper. Place fish in the pan and cook for 5–6 minutes until opaque. Mix in cilantro before serving.

PER SERVING: Calories: 157 | GI: Very low | Carbohydrates: 7g | Protein: 19g | Fat: 7g

CHAPTER 14

Dressings and Sauces

Country Barbecue Sauce

You can change the flavor of this sauce by adding
a chopped lemon, orange juice, or lime juice.

INGREDIENTS | MAKES 1 QUART (8 SERVINGS)

4 cloves garlic, chopped

2 large yellow onions, chopped

2 sweet red peppers, chopped

2 serrano chili peppers, cored, seeded, and minced (optional)

2 tablespoons olive oil

1 teaspoon salt, or to taste

2 teaspoons black pepper

1 teaspoon Tabasco sauce, or to taste

2 ounces cider vinegar

2 tablespoons Dijon-style prepared mustard

1 28-ounce can tomato purée

2 tablespoons molasses

1 teaspoon liquid smoke

4 whole cloves

1 cinnamon stick

1 teaspoon hot paprika

1 tablespoon sweet paprika

1. In a large soup pot, sauté the garlic, onions, and peppers in olive oil. Stirring constantly, add the rest of the ingredients. Bring to a boil. Reduce heat.

2. Cover the pot and simmer for 2 hours. If you don't like the texture, purée in a blender.

PER SERVING (4 OUNCES): Calories: 118 | GI: Very low | Carbohydrates: 18g | Protein: 3g | Fat: 4g

Sweet, Spicy, or Both

The amount of heat you add to barbecue sauce is a matter of personal taste, as is the amount of sweetness. Some people prefer the flavor of honey over molasses; others use brown sugar. Experiment!

Yogurt and Herb (Ranch) Dressing

This is delicious with vegetables.

INGREDIENTS | MAKES 1 CUP
(8 SERVINGS)

7 ounces low-fat yogurt
2 tablespoons lemon juice
2 tablespoons chives, chopped
½ teaspoon celery salt
½ teaspoon garlic powder
2 drops Tabasco sauce, or to taste

Whisk all ingredients together and serve.

PER SERVING (2 TABLESPOONS): Calories: 17 | GI: Very low | Carbohydrates: 2g | Protein: 1g | Fat: 0g

Caesar Dressing

True Caesar salad dressing has a touch of anchovy, lemon, and mustard.

INGREDIENTS | MAKES 1 CUP
(8 SERVINGS)

¼ cup red wine vinegar
1 raw (pasteurized) egg
1 clove garlic, mashed
1 tablespoon lemon juice
½ teaspoon dry English mustard
½" anchovy paste
Salt and pepper, to taste
¼ cup Parmesan cheese, freshly grated
¼ cup olive oil
Garnish of parsley, to taste

1. In the blender, blend the vinegar, egg, garlic, and lemon juice until puréed. Add the mustard, anchovy paste, salt, pepper, and cheese.

2. With the blender running on medium speed, slowly pour in the olive oil in a thin stream. Garnish with fresh parsley, to taste.

Which Olive Oil Is Best?

Extra-virgin olive oil comes from the first pressing of the olives, has the most intense flavor, and is the most expensive. Use this for salads and for dressings and dips. Virgin olive oil is from the second pressing. Less expensive than extra-virgin, it can be used for the same purposes. "Olive oil" indicates that it is from the last pressing; this is the oil used for cooking since it does not burn as easily at high temperatures.

PER SERVING (1 OUNCE): Calories: 83 | GI: Zero | Carbohydrates: 0g | Protein: 2g | Fat: 9g

Lemon Pepper Dressing

Peppercorns and chilies offer different flavors in cooking. Peppercorns are dried berries, and chilies are the hot fruit of a plant and have spicy seeds. This recipe is a wonderful marriage of pepper flavors. Use it with grilled vegetables, as well as on salads.

INGREDIENTS | MAKES 1 CUP (8 SERVINGS)

7 ounces low-fat mayonnaise

Juice and minced rind of ½ lemon

1 teaspoon Dijon-style mustard

1 teaspoon freshly ground black pepper

½ teaspoon white pepper

½ teaspoon red pepper flakes

Salt, to taste

¼ teaspoon anchovy paste

Whisk all ingredients together and serve with chicken, salad, or cold meats.

PER SERVING (1 OUNCE): Calories: 81 | GI: Zero | Carbohydrates: 2g | Protein: 0g | Fat: 8g

Hollandaise Sauce

If you make hollandaise sauce in the blender or food processor, your sauce will not curdle.

INGREDIENTS | MAKES ¾ CUP (6 SERVINGS)

4 ounces sweet unsalted butter

1 whole egg

1 egg yolk

¼ teaspoon dry mustard

Juice of ½ lemon

⅛ teaspoon cayenne pepper

Salt, to taste

1. Melt the butter over very low heat. While the butter is melting, blend all but the salt in the blender or food processor.

2. With the blender running on medium speed, slowly add the butter, a little at a time. Return the sauce to a low heat and whisk until thickened. Add salt and serve immediately.

TIP: *Substitute vegan butter for regular butter to cut back on saturated fat.*

PER SERVING (1 OUNCE): Calories: 161 | GI: Zero | Carbohydrates: 0g | Protein: 2g | Fat: 17g

Béarnaise Sauce and Sauce Maltaise

If you substitute white wine vinegar for lemon juice and add chives in this recipe, you will have béarnaise sauce, a classic for steaks. If you substitute orange juice (preferably from a blood orange) for lemon juice, you'll have Sauce Maltaise, which is delicious with vegetables.

Horseradish Sauce

This is a classic with corned beef. It can be used for hot or cold meats, fish, or seafood.
When you see rosy horseradish in the supermarket, try it.
Rosy horseradish is colored and slightly sweetened with beet juice.

INGREDIENTS | MAKES 1 CUP
(8 SERVINGS)

1 cup low-fat sour cream

1 tablespoon prepared horseradish

1 tablespoon lemon juice

Salt and freshly ground black pepper, to taste

Using a fork, mix all ingredients together in a bowl and serve.

PER SERVING (1 OUNCE): Calories: 32 | GI: Very low | Carbohydrates: 1g | Protein: 0g | Fat: 3g

Sweet and Sour Dressing

You can use this as a dressing for salad, especially Asian noodle salads, or hot noodles.
You can also use it on pork, chicken, or beef.

INGREDIENTS | MAKES ½ CUP
(8 SERVINGS)

3 ounces soy sauce

1 teaspoon Asian sesame seed oil

1 teaspoon fresh ginger, minced

1 tablespoon maple syrup or honey

1 tablespoon concentrated orange juice

1 tablespoon apricot preserves or jam

1 clove garlic, minced

1 teaspoon Tabasco sauce, or to taste

Whisk all ingredients together over low heat until well blended and serve.

PER SERVING (1 TABLESPOON): Calories: 22 | GI: Low | Carbohydrates: 4g | Protein: 0g | Fat: 1g

Mustard Cream Sauce (Hot)

This is a perfect complement to chicken, goose, duck, or veal.

INGREDIENTS | SERVES 4

2 tablespoons olive oil

2 shallots, minced

1 clove garlic, minced

1 teaspoon flour

⅔ cup chicken broth

1 ounce dry vermouth

1 tablespoon Dijon-style mustard, prepared

2 ounces heavy cream

Salt and pepper, to taste

1. Heat the olive oil over medium flame. Add the shallots and garlic; sauté for 5 minutes or until soft. Whisk in the flour and cook for another 2–3 minutes. Whisk in the chicken broth, vermouth, and mustard.

2. Bring the sauce to a boil. Whisk in the cream and turn off heat. Taste for salt and pepper and add accordingly.

PER SERVING (2 OUNCES): Calories: 111 | GI: Very low | Carbohydrates: 1g | Protein: 0g | Fat: 0g

Aioli

Aioli is a basic French mayonnaise used throughout the Mediterranean.
It's loaded with garlic and can have a variety of different herbs. You can add tomatoes and spices.

INGREDIENTS | MAKES 1 CUP
(16 SERVINGS)

2 pasteurized eggs, at room temperature

1 teaspoon lemon juice

1 teaspoon white wine vinegar

½ teaspoon Dijon-style mustard

4 cloves garlic, or to taste

¾ cup olive oil

Choice of ½ teaspoon oregano, tarragon, or rosemary

Salt and pepper, to taste

1. Place the eggs, lemon juice, vinegar, mustard, and garlic in the blender.

2. Add the olive oil a little at a time. When the mixture is creamy, taste; add herbs, salt, and pepper. Pulse to blend; store in the refrigerator or serve.

PER SERVING (1 TABLESPOON): Calories: 99 | GI: Zero | Carbohydrates: 0g | Protein: 1g

Storing Aioli

Aioli will keep in the refrigerator for a day or two, but it's best made and used the same day.

Green Olive Sauce

This is a wonderful garnish or spread for a good hot Tuscan bread.
There is no salt in this recipe because the olives are very salty.

INGREDIENTS | MAKES 1 CUP
(8 SERVINGS)

⅔ cup green olives, pitted and chopped

½ cup fresh parsley

Juice of ½ lemon

Rind of ½ lemon, minced

1 tablespoon chives, minced, fresh only

1 cup cream cheese, at room temperature

Freshly ground black pepper, to taste

Mix all ingredients together. Chill for 2 hours. Serve at room temperature.

TIP: *You can substitute low-fat cream cheese for regular cream cheese in this spread.*

PER SERVING (2 TABLESPOONS): Calories: 85 | GI: Very low | Carbohydrates: 0g | Protein: 1g | Fat: 5g

Grilled Peach Chutney

Grilled fruit is wonderful with any number of meats, poultry, or fish.
Grilled peach chutney is sublime!

INGREDIENTS | MAKES 2 CUPS
(16 SERVINGS)

6 medium-sized freestone peaches, halved and pitted

½ red onion, minced

2 jalapeño peppers, cored, seeded, and minced

Juice of 1 lime

½ teaspoon ground cloves

½ teaspoon ground allspice

½ teaspoon coriander seeds, ground

½ cup light brown sugar, or to taste

¼ cup white wine vinegar

1 teaspoon salt, or to taste

Freshly ground black pepper, to taste

Red pepper flakes, to taste

¼ bunch fresh cilantro, chopped

1. Grill the peaches, cut-side down, over low flame until they are soft but not falling apart, about 5 minutes.

2. Cool them and then slip off the skins. Using a knife, cut them into chunks and place in a bowl. This method retains the juice and some texture.

3. Mix the rest of the ingredients into the bowl with the peaches. Cool, cover, and refrigerate until ready to serve. Warm just before serving.

PER SERVING (2 TABLESPOONS): Calories: 45 | GI: Very low | Carbohydrates: 12g | Protein: 0g | Fat: 0g

Fresh Tomato Dressing

This is perfect over shrimp, drizzled onto avocados, or even used as a sauce
for hot or cold chicken or fish. It tastes summery!

INGREDIENTS | MAKES 2 CUPS
(16 SERVINGS)

1 pint cherry tomatoes

4 cloves roasted garlic

2 shallots

2 jalapeño peppers, cored and seeded

¼ cup stemmed, loosely packed fresh basil

¼ cup red wine or balsamic vinegar

½ cup extra-virgin olive oil

½ teaspoon celery salt

2 teaspoons Worcestershire sauce

Freshly ground black pepper, to taste

½ teaspoon cayenne pepper, or to taste

Purée all ingredients in the blender. Taste for salt and pepper. This dressing improves with age—try making it a day or two in advance.

PER SERVING (2 TABLESPOONS): Calories: 78 | GI: Very low | Carbohydrates: 2g | Protein: 0g | Fat: 7g

Balsamic Vinegar

There are various types of Italian vinegar, but perhaps the most famous is balsamic vinegar. Balsamic vinegar is made from reduced wine and aged in special wood barrels for years. Each year's barrels are made of a different type of wood—the vinegar absorbs the flavor of the wood. Authentic balsamic vinegar ages for a minimum of 10 and up to 30 years.

Caramelized Onions

*These are wonderful on everything from sandwiches
to salads and as a garnish for roasts and stews.*

INGREDIENTS | MAKES 1 CUP

3 large Vidalia or other sweet onions,
sliced ⅛" thick
1 tablespoon olive oil

Timesaving Tip

This recipe can be made ahead of time and
kept on hand in a small glass jar for 3–5
days to use as a condiment and add flavor
to many lunch and dinner dishes.

Place the onions in a large sauté pan with olive oil.
Over very low heat, sauté for 20 minutes, or until
onions are browned but not burned.

PER SERVING: Calories: 420 | GI: Very low | Carbohydrates:
75g | Protein: 9g | Fat: 12g

Pomegranate Sauce

*This is excellent with game or any kind of poultry.
Try it with grilled or roasted venison.*

INGREDIENTS | MAKES 1 CUP
(8 SERVINGS)

1½ cups pomegranate juice
½ cup sugar substitute
Juice and rind of ½ orange, seeded
2 whole cloves

Mix all ingredients in a saucepan. Bring to a boil.
Reduce heat and simmer until reduced to 1 cup. Its
consistency should be syrupy.

PER SERVING: Calories: 30 | GI: Moderate | Carbohydrates:
11g | Protein: 0g | Fat: 0g

Cucumber, Dill, and Sour Cream Sauce

*This recipe is marvelous with poached, chilled salmon.
Use fresh herbs only!*

**INGREDIENTS | MAKES 2 CUPS, SERVES 4
AS A SAUCE/DRESSING**

1½ cups cucumber, peeled and chopped
½ cup red onion, finely chopped
Juice of 1 lemon
1 teaspoon Tabasco sauce
½ cup low-fat sour cream
1 teaspoon celery salt, or to taste
½ cup fresh dill, finely minced
2 tablespoons minced chives
½ teaspoon sweet paprika, or to taste

Mix all ingredients in a bowl. Cover and refrigerate for 1 hour. Serve chilled.

PER SERVING: Calories: 62 | GI: Very low | Carbohydrates: 10g | Protein: 1g | Fat: 4g

Roasted Garlic

*This is useful as a spread for bread and as an addition
to salad dressings and marinades.*

INGREDIENTS | MAKES 1 HEAD GARLIC

1 head garlic
1 teaspoon olive oil
2 tablespoons water

The Power of Garlic

Although it may not protect against vampires, garlic is known for possessing numerous health-promoting properties. Fresh garlic contains anti-inflammatory compounds that may help reduce inflammation-related conditions from arthritis pain to heart attacks. The antibacterial and antiviral properties of garlic have been studied extensively. So pile on the garlic for flavor and good health.

1. Preheat oven to 350°F. Cut off top of garlic, ¼" down.

2. Make a pocket with aluminum foil and add garlic, olive oil, and water. Roast for 1 hour.

3. Separate individual cloves. Squeeze over bread, into dressings, or add to a variety of marinades.

PER SERVING: Calories: 40 | GI: Zero | Carbohydrates: 0g | Protein: 0g | Fat: 5g

Salsa Verde

Tomatillos, a relative of the tomato, are in peak season in the summer and early autumn.

INGREDIENTS | MAKES 3 CUPS

1½ pounds fresh tomatillos

2 jalapeño peppers

½ cup fresh cilantro, chopped

1 onion, chopped

Juice of 1 lime

2 teaspoons salt

1. Preheat oven to 400°F. Remove husks from the tomatillos, rinse in warm water, and place on a baking sheet. Place jalapeños and tomatillos in the oven to roast until slightly charred, about 10 minutes.

2. Place tomatillos, jalapeños, cilantro, onion, lime juice, and salt in a blender. Purée until salsa is well-blended.

PER SERVING (¼ CUP): Calories: 23 | GI: Very low | Carbohydrates: 5g | Protein: 1g | Fat: 1g

Cajun Rémoulade

This spicy sauce pairs well with seafood dishes, adding zest and a bit of heat.

INGREDIENTS | MAKES ABOUT 2 CUPS

3 tablespoons lemon juice

1 cup low-fat plain Greek yogurt

¼ large onion, minced

4 green onions, chopped

3 cloves garlic, minced

1½ tablespoons horseradish

1 tablespoon relish

2 tablespoons Dijon mustard

2 tablespoons tomato paste

½ teaspoon salt

Cayenne and black pepper, to taste

Mix all ingredients in a bowl using a fork or a food processor.

PER SERVING (2 TABLESPOONS): Calories: 17 | GI: Very low | Carbohydrates: 3g | Protein: 1g | Fat: 0g

Fresh Tomato Sauce for Steak or Chicken

This is a very versatile sauce—use it on any meat or poultry.

INGREDIENTS | MAKES ⅔ CUP (SERVES 2)

3 large fresh tomatoes

1 quart boiling water

2 cloves garlic, chopped

Salt and pepper, to taste

1 teaspoon Worcestershire sauce

2 tablespoons parsley, chopped

Blanch the tomatoes in boiling water, drain, slip off skins, and chop. In a small bowl, mix the chopped tomatoes with the rest of the ingredients. Serve warm.

PER SERVING: Calories: 44 | GI: Very low | Carbohydrates: 10g | Protein: 2g | Fat: 0g

Sour Cream Chive Sauce

This is a rich, creamy, and spicy sauce.

INGREDIENTS | MAKES ½ CUP (SERVES 4)

½ cup sour cream

¼ cup chives, snipped fine with kitchen shears

1 teaspoon prepared horseradish, or to taste

Salt and pepper, to taste

Mix all ingredients in a small bowl; serve chilled.

TIP: *You can replace the sour cream in this sauce with low-fat sour cream.*

PER SERVING: Calories: 62 | GI: Zero | Carbohydrates: 2g | Protein: 0g | Fat: 6g

Mint Chimichurri Sauce

Instead of the traditional mint jelly,
use this mint chimichurri sauce to make a lamb recipe extra special.

INGREDIENTS | MAKES 2 CUPS

2 cups fresh parsley

2 cups fresh cilantro

1 cup fresh mint

¾ cup olive oil

3 tablespoons red wine vinegar

Juice of 1 lemon

3 cloves garlic, minced

1 large shallot, quartered

1 teaspoon salt

1 small jalapeño, seeded and chopped

1. Wash herbs, remove stems, and chop leaves.

2. In a blender, add olive oil, vinegar, lemon juice, garlic, shallots, salt, and jalapeño; blend ingredients together. Add parsley, cilantro, and mint to the blender in batches and blend until sauce is smooth.

PER SERVING (2 TABLESPOONS): Calories: 98 | GI: Very low | Carbohydrates: 2g | Protein: 0g | Fat: 10g

CHAPTER 15

Side Dishes

Celeriac Slaw for Garnish or Appetizers

In France, celeriac (a vegetable in the celery family) is used at cocktail time on a toasted piece of baguette, dressed with a shrimp, a mussel, or some other delicious treat. You can put this slaw next to most meat, fish, or poultry for a tasty counterpoint.

INGREDIENTS | MAKES ⅔ CUP (6 SERVINGS)

1 celeriac bulb, peeled and coarsely grated
1 tablespoon low-fat mayonnaise
1 tablespoon white wine vinegar
Pinch dried thyme
Salt and pepper, to taste
1 teaspoon dry English mustard

Place the celeriac in a bowl. In a separate bowl, mix mayonnaise, vinegar, thyme, salt, pepper, and mustard. Pour over the celeriac and serve as a garnish or as part of an appetizer tray.

PER SERVING: Calories: 45 | GI: Zero | Carbohydrates: 9g | Protein: 1g | Fat: 1g

Baked Sweet Potato Sticks

These fries are good for you and make a delicious and energizing side dish that substitutes for traditional French fries. Great for kids!

INGREDIENTS | 1 LARGE POTATO SERVES 2

1 large sweet potato, peeled, cut like French fries
1 tablespoon olive oil
Salt and pepper, to taste
1 teaspoon thyme leaves, dried
1 teaspoon sage leaves, dried

1. Blanch the peeled potato slices in boiling water for 4–5 minutes. Dry on paper towels.

2. Sprinkle with olive oil, salt, pepper, and herbs. Bake in an aluminum pan at 350°F until crisp, about 10 minutes.

PER SERVING: Calories: 104 | GI: Moderate | Carbohydrates: 21g | Protein: 2g | Fat: 2g

Sweet Potato Benefits

Full of fiber, potassium, and beta-carotene, sweet potatoes are an often-neglected healthy and delicious vegetable—most people forget about them until Thanksgiving! Their bright orange flesh adds color to any meal, they can be cooked like regular potatoes, and they taste best when baked.

Napa Cabbage with Asian Sauce

You can use napa cabbage (cooked or raw) instead of pasta as a bed for sauces and meats and as a salad green. Try it steamed with various sauces. It is very low on the GI and adds fiber and antioxidants. This sauce can be adapted to your taste, from fruity to hot.

INGREDIENTS | SERVES 2

¼ cup peanut oil

2 tablespoons sesame seed oil

6 scallions

1" gingerroot, peeled and minced

1 clove garlic, minced

½ cup soy sauce

½ napa cabbage, cut crosswise in thin slices, separated into ribbons

Heat the oils and sauté the scallions, gingerroot, and garlic. Add the soy sauce and garnish. Rinse the cabbage and drain on paper towels; toss with Asian sauce.

PER SERVING: Calories: 90 | GI: Zero | Carbohydrates: 7g | Protein: 5g | Fat: 4g

Asian-Style Garnishes

To add flair to the presentation of this dish, try topping it with 1 tablespoon toasted sesame seeds and a squeeze of the juice of half a lime. Serve with lime wedges and chopsticks.

Quinoa with Lime and Mint

This is a fresh and zesty quinoa dish that pairs well with boldly seasoned grilled meats and fish.

INGREDIENTS | SERVES 4

2½ cups water

1 cup quinoa, uncooked

2 tablespoons olive oil

Juice from 1 lime

½ teaspoon lime zest

2 tablespoons fresh mint, chopped

1 clove garlic, minced

1 red bell pepper, diced

Salt and pepper, to taste

1. Pour water into a small pot or rice cooker; add quinoa, cover, and cook 20 minutes or until the quinoa is tender and all the water is absorbed.

2. Transfer quinoa to a mixing bowl and add olive oil, lime juice, lime zest, mint, garlic, and bell pepper; stir to combine. Season quinoa with salt and pepper as desired.

3. Serve chilled.

PER SERVING: Calories: 230 | GI: Moderate | Carbohydrates: 30g | Protein: 6g | Fat: 9g

Roasted Broccoli with Lemon and Romano Cheese

For a gourmet twist try replacing broccoli florets with broccoli rabe or broccolini.

INGREDIENTS | SERVES 4

4 cups raw broccoli florets

3 tablespoons olive oil

Salt and pepper, to taste

¾ cup Romano cheese, grated

Juice of 1 lemon

1. Heat oven to 400°F.

2. Place broccoli in a large glass baking dish, drizzle with oil, and season with salt and pepper as desired. Place broccoli in the oven and roast for 12 minutes.

3. Remove broccoli from the oven and cover the top evenly with cheese and lemon juice. Return the broccoli to the oven and cook until cheese is melted, about 10 minutes.

PER SERVING: Calories: 222 | GI: Low | Carbohydrates: 6g | Protein: 11g | Fat: 18g

German-Style Potato Salad

This recipe is exceptionally flavorful and tasty and is wonderful when served with barbecued meats.

INGREDIENTS | SERVES 4

2 large Idaho, russet, or Yukon gold potatoes

¼ cup cider vinegar

¼ cup vegetable oil

1 teaspoon salt

1 teaspoon pepper

1 teaspoon sugar

1 teaspoon Hungarian sweet paprika

1 red onion, chopped

2 scallions, chopped

½ cup fresh parsley, chopped

1. Peel potatoes and cut into ½" slices.

2. Boil the potatoes in salted water to cover, 10–15 minutes, or until just softened.

3. Mix the rest of the ingredients in a large bowl. Drain potatoes and add to the dressing immediately. Toss gently to coat. Serve hot or cold.

PER SERVING: Calories: 257 | GI: Medium | Carbohydrates: 32g | Protein: 4g | Fat: 14g

Old-Town Cole Slaw

Too much mayonnaise makes cole slaw heavy.
Try this Baltimore recipe that is a little lighter on the mayonnaise than traditional slaw recipes.

INGREDIENTS | SERVES 4

¼ cup cider vinegar

1 teaspoon sugar

¼ cup low-fat mayonnaise

¼ teaspoon celery salt

Freshly ground black pepper, to taste

¼ teaspoon celery seeds

3 cups shredded cabbage

½ cup red onion, shredded

Mix the first six ingredients in a large bowl. Add the cabbage and onions. Chill for 1 hour and serve.

PER SERVING: Calories: 67 | GI: Zero | Carbohydrates: 6g | Protein: 1g | Fat: 5g

Cole Slaw History

Food historians believe that the modern cole slaw recipe has actually been around for at least 200 years. Today cole slaw is served with barbecue, burgers, chicken, and other cooked foods. Shredded carrots and a mix of red and green cabbage can be used to make cole slaw colorful and fun.

Baked Spaghetti Squash

Spaghetti squash gets its name from the long, noodle-like strands of flesh that can be scraped away from the shell of a cooked squash.

INGREDIENTS | SERVES 4

1 spaghetti squash
2 tablespoons olive oil
⅓ cup Parmesan cheese, grated
Salt and pepper, to taste

1. Slice squash in half lengthwise and remove seeds and fibers with a large spoon. Place the squash in a baking dish and with water to cover the bottom of the dish.

2. Bake at 350°F for 1 hour until tender. Remove from baking dish and let cool for 15 minutes.

3. Scrape the inside flesh out and place in a serving bowl. Mix with olive oil, Parmesan cheese, and salt and pepper as desired.

PER SERVING: Calories: 133 | GI: Low | Carbohydrates: 16g | Protein: 4g | Fat: 7g

Cranberry Ring with Walnut, Celeriac, Dried Cranberry, and Apple Salad

This is another old-fashioned dish, adapted for modern tables.

INGREDIENTS | SERVES 8

2 envelopes unflavored gelatin

1 cup 100% cranberry juice, sugar-free, cold

2 cups cranberry juice cocktail, sugar-free, heated

1 teaspoon Tabasco sauce

¼ cup orange juice

2 tart apples, peeled, cored, and chopped

½ cup walnuts, toasted, chopped

1 whole celeriac root, peeled and grated

½ cup dried cranberries

¼ cup white wine vinegar

1 cup low-fat mayonnaise

1. Place the gelatin in the bowl of a blender. Cover with ¼ cup cold cranberry juice and allow to bloom for 5 minutes, expanding and softening. With the blender running on medium speed, add the hot cranberry juice cocktail, Tabasco sauce, the remaining cold cranberry juice, and orange juice. Pour into a 1½ quart ring mold.

2. Add 1 apple. Refrigerate until set, about 2 hours.

3. Make the salad by mixing the second apple, walnuts, celeriac, dried cranberries, vinegar, and mayonnaise together. When ready to serve, turn the ring onto a platter and surround it with the salad.

PER SERVING: Calories: 315 | GI: Low | Carbohydrates: 38g | Protein: 5g | Fat: 18g

Wild Rice Casserole with Hazelnuts and Dried Apricots

*This rice dish has a hint of fruity sweetness from the apricots that
will make it a standout side dish at your holiday table.*

INGREDIENTS | SERVES 8

4 cups water

1 cup wild rice

1 teaspoon salt, or to taste

½ sweet onion, such as Vidalia, chopped

1 tablespoon butter, plus 2 teaspoons

1 cup dried apricots, cut into pieces

1 cup chicken broth

½ cup hazelnuts, toasted

½ cup baked ham, finely chopped

Freshly ground black pepper, to taste

Wild Rice Basics

When cooking wild rice, always use more liquid than the recipe on the box suggests. Wild rice should fully bloom, not be tiny spikes when cooked.

1. Bring the water to a boil; add the wild rice and salt. Reduce heat; cover and simmer for 1 hour or until grains are fully opened.

2. Sauté the onion in 1 tablespoon butter. In a separate bowl, cover the apricots with chicken broth and allow to expand for 30 minutes. When the rice is fully cooked, place in a casserole dish. Add the sautéed onions, apricots soaked in broth, nuts, baked ham, and pepper.

3. Dot with 2 teaspoons butter and bake for 15 minutes at 250°F, letting the flavors blend.

TIP: *Substitute heart-healthy margarine or olive oil for butter in this casserole.*

PER SERVING: Calories: 183 | GI: Moderate | Carbohydrates: 22g | Protein: 6g | Fat: 10g

Fresh Corn Stuffing for Poultry, Fish, or Game

Stuffing can be piled on top of a dish instead of being stuffed into meat. This dish is exceptional, a remembrance of the first Thanksgiving and the Native Americans' gift of corn to the starving Pilgrims.

INGREDIENTS | MAKES 4 CUPS

¼ pound butter or margarine

1 sweet medium-sized onion, chopped

4 celery stalks with leaves, chopped

1 cup chicken, vegetable, or beef stock (depending on what you're stuffing)

20 juniper berries, bruised

1 teaspoon dried thyme, or 1 tablespoon fresh

1 teaspoon dried savory, or 1 tablespoon fresh

1 teaspoon dried sage, or 1 tablespoon fresh

½ cup fresh parsley, chopped

2 cups cornbread stuffing, from a package

2 cups frozen corn

1 cup 2% milk

1. Melt the butter or margarine in a pan over medium heat. Sauté the onions and celery for 5–7 minutes.

2. Add the broth, juniper berries, herbs, and spices. Mix well and add the cornbread stuffing, corn, and milk. Use with any holiday entrée.

> **TIP:** *To lower the fat and calories of this recipe, substitute heart-healthy margarine or olive oil for butter; replace 2% milk with nonfat milk; and you can replace the sour cream in this sauce with low-fat sour cream.*

PER SERVING (1 CUP): Calories: 460 | GI: Moderate | Carbohydrates: 48g | Protein: 8g | Fat: 26g

Twice-Baked Sweet Potatoes

These sweet potatoes are not just for holidays; they should be enjoyed year-round.

INGREDIENTS | SERVES 4

4 sweet potatoes
2 tablespoons butter, softened
3 ounces low-fat cream cheese
1 tablespoon agave nectar
¼ teaspoon cinnamon
¼ teaspoon ginger

1. Preheat oven to 375°F.

2. Wash sweet potatoes and then place on a baking sheet. Bake for 1 hour. Allow potatoes to cool. Slice potatoes in half lengthwise and scoop out inside flesh into a mixing bowl. Keep potato skins intact.

3. In a second mixing bowl, combine butter, cream cheese, agave nectar, and spices. Add the cream cheese mixture to the sweet potato and mash to blend well.

4. Fill the potato skins with the sweet potato mash and place on a baking sheet. Place in the oven to bake for 15 minutes.

PER SERVING: Calories: 206 | GI: Low | Carbohydrates: 28g | Protein: 4g | Fat: 9g

Brussels Sprouts Hash with Caramelized Shallots

Even those who dislike Brussels sprouts will gobble this up.

INGREDIENTS | SERVES 6

1 pound Brussels sprouts

2 shallots, thinly sliced

¼ cup olive oil

Salt and pepper, to taste

3 tablespoons balsamic vinegar

1. Trim stems off Brussels sprouts and slice in half lengthwise. Place Brussels sprouts and shallots in a shallow baking dish. Coat Brussels sprouts with olive oil; season with salt and pepper as desired.

2. Bake for 20 minutes at 400°F. Remove dish from the oven, and drizzle vinegar evenly over Brussels sprouts. Return dish to the oven to bake for 3–4 minutes.

PER SERVING: Calories: 121 | GI: Very low | Carbohydrates: 9g | Protein: 3g | Fat: 9g

Moroccan Couscous with Apricots

Couscous is very small pasta, popular in Morocco and other areas of the Middle East.
It cooks quickly, lends itself to many dishes, and is a good substitute for rice.

INGREDIENTS | SERVES 4

8 ounces dried apricots

2 cups hot water

1 tablespoon sugar

1 cup couscous

1½ cups boiling water

Juice and rind of ½ lemon

½ teaspoon coriander seeds, ground

1 teaspoon dried sage leaves, crumbled,
or 1 tablespoon fresh sage, torn

1 tablespoon butter

1 teaspoon salt, or to taste

1. Cut the apricots in quarters and soak in 2 cups hot water with sugar for 1 hour.

2. Stir the couscous into the boiling water. Add apricots, lemon juice, and lemon rind.

3. Cook, stirring, until water has absorbed. Add coriander and sage.

4. Stir in butter and salt. Serve hot or warm.

TIP: *In this couscous recipe, you can substitute olive oil or heart-healthy margarine for butter.*

Couscous Variety

Couscous is unique because it is equally delicious with both fruits and vegetables, working well as a sweet or savory dish or even as a sweet-savory dish.

PER SERVING: Calories: 328 | GI: Very low | Carbohydrates: 67g | Protein: 8g | Fat: 4g

Tofu with Shrimp and Vegetables

Almost any dish can be pepped up with hot pepper sauce, lemon zest,
lemon or lime juice, or aromatic herbs. Try making any basic sauce and throw in any of these.
Keep tasting until you get more zip! This is a basic stir-fry with a kick.

INGREDIENTS | SERVES 2

2 teaspoons peanut oil

1 teaspoon Asian sesame oil

1 teaspoon fresh gingerroot, peeled and minced

1 cup bean sprouts

1 cup sugar snap peas

1 teaspoon tahini

4 ounces satin tofu

6 ounces small shrimp, peeled and deveined

1 tablespoon soy sauce

1 teaspoon Thai chili paste, or red hot pepper sauce

1. Heat oils in a wok or nonstick pan over medium-high heat.

2. Stir in the ginger, bean sprouts, and snap peas. Stir and cook for 2 minutes.

3. Add the rest of the ingredients, stirring until shrimp turns pink. Serve immediately.

PER SERVING: Calories: 270 | GI: Zero | Carbohydrates: 14g | Protein: 29g | Fat: 13g

Types of Tofu

Tofu is a versatile food that comes in a few different types, all of which are low in calories and high in protein. Firm tofu is best for grilling, whereas soft tofu is suitable for blended dishes or soups. Satin or silken tofu is more creamy and custard-like but does come in extra-firm varieties that you can stir-fry.

Mashed Cauliflower

A healthier alternative to mashed potatoes, mashed cauliflower is lower in calories, fat, and carbohydrates.

INGREDIENTS | SERVES 6

1 head cauliflower
2 tablespoons olive oil
1 tablespoon fresh chives, chopped
Salt and pepper, to taste

1. Place cauliflower in a large pot of boiling water, and cook for 10 minutes. Drain well, reserving ¼ cup boiling liquid.

2. Place cauliflower in blender or food processor with oil and cooking liquid and purée until smooth. Add chives and season with salt and pepper as desired.

PER SERVING: Calories: 95 | GI: Very low | Carbohydrates: 7g | Protein: 3g | Fat: 7g

Baked Polenta Fries

These fries go over well at parties. Serve hot with a variety of dipping sauces.

INGREDIENTS | SERVES 6

2 cups low-fat milk
2 cups water
1½ cups polenta
1 teaspoon salt, plus more to taste
½ cup Parmesan cheese, grated
3 tablespoons olive oil

1. Add milk and water to a saucepan and bring to a boil. While stirring, add polenta to the pan. Turn the heat down to medium. Add 1 teaspoon salt and Parmesan. Cook and stir until polenta thickens.

2. Remove the pan from the heat. Spread the polenta out onto a baking sheet, about ½" thick. Place baking sheet in the refrigerator for 1 hour.

3. Remove polenta from the refrigerator and cut into large fry-shaped pieces. Rub them with olive oil and sprinkle with salt, as desired.

4. Bake at 450°F for 10 minutes on each side. Fries should be golden brown and crispy.

PER SERVING: Calories: 318 | GI: Moderate | Carbohydrates: 45g | Protein: 10g | Fat: 11g

Quinoa and Black Beans

Although it looks like grain or rice, quinoa is technically a seed.
It is rich in protein, fiber, and iron.

INGREDIENTS | SERVES 6

2 teaspoons olive oil

1 medium onion, chopped

1 cup white mushrooms, sliced

3 cloves garlic, chopped

¾ cup quinoa, uncooked

1½ cups chicken broth

¼ teaspoon crushed red pepper

Salt and pepper, to taste

1 15-ounce can black beans, drained and rinsed

¼ cup cilantro, chopped

1. Add oil to medium saucepan over medium heat. Add onion, mushrooms, and garlic to hot pan; sauté for 5 minutes.

2. Rinse quinoa with cool water for 1–2 minutes. Add quinoa to the saucepan along with broth. Season with crushed red pepper; add salt and pepper as desired.

3. Bring to a boil, then cover, reduce heat to low, and simmer for 20 minutes.

4. Mix beans into the quinoa and cook for 4–5 minutes. Serve and garnish with cilantro.

PER SERVING: Calories: 199 | GI: Moderate | Carbohydrates: 30g | Protein: 12g | Fat: 4g

Mixed Beans in Vinaigrette

This simple side can be made ahead for last-minute time savings.

INGREDIENTS | SERVES 12

½ pound bacon
1 tablespoon agave nectar
1 teaspoon salt
¼ teaspoon pepper
¾ cup red wine vinegar
½ cup water
½ pound green beans
½ pound yellow wax beans
1 15-ounce can kidney beans
1 15-ounce can navy beans
1 15-ounce can chickpeas

1. Chop bacon into small pieces and place in a large pan over medium-high heat. Cook bacon, stirring frequently with a slotted spoon, until browned. Remove bacon from the pan, leaving behind excess oil. Set bacon aside.

2. Add agave nectar, salt, and pepper to bacon drippings in the pan and stir. Add in vinegar and water; bring to a boil while continuing to stir. Cover pan and reduce heat to low; simmer for 10 minutes.

3. Meanwhile, steam green and yellow beans until crisp-tender. Drain, and place in a large serving bowl. Rinse canned beans and pour into the same bowl.

4. Toss the mixed beans with warm vinaigrette, and sprinkle with bacon crumbles.

PER SERVING: Calories: 253 | GI: Low | Carbohydrates: 29g | Protein: 11g | Fat: 11g

Warm Red Cabbage with Goat Cheese and Bacon

With so many dominant flavors, this delicious side can even stand on its own as a lunch.

INGREDIENTS | SERVES 6

1 head red cabbage
¼ pound bacon, chopped
2 tablespoons olive oil
3 tablespoons balsamic vinegar
2 cloves garlic, minced
¼ teaspoon pepper
5 ounces goat cheese

1. Slice cabbage head in half, remove the core, and chop into small pieces.

2. In a large pan over medium-high heat, cook bacon pieces until browned and crisp. Drain excess oil from the pan. Place cabbage into pan with bacon.

3. Add oil, vinegar, garlic, and pepper to the cabbage. Cover, reduce heat to low, and simmer for 10 minutes, until tender.

4. Toss cabbage with goat cheese and serve.

PER SERVING: Calories: 255 | GI: Low | Carbohydrates: 16g | Protein: 9g | Fat: 18g

Sicilian-Style Radishes and Tuna

The secret to a tasty and pleasing final result is using a good quality water-packed tuna.

INGREDIENTS | SERVES 2

1 bunch radishes
1 can albacore tuna, drained
1 tablespoon red wine vinegar
Juice of ½ lemon
1 teaspoon olive oil
1 teaspoon chives, chopped
Salt and pepper, to taste
2 large romaine or butter lettuce leaves

1. Slice leaves away from radishes and clean well. Cut radishes into ¼"-thick slices.

2. Using a fork, place tuna in a medium bowl, allowing tuna to remain in chunks. Add radishes, vinegar, lemon juice, oil, chives, salt, and pepper to the tuna and stir to combine.

3. Serve on a leaf of lettuce.

PER SERVING: Calories: 121 | GI: Very low | Carbohydrates: 2g | Protein: 21g | Fat: 5g

CHAPTER 16

Desserts

Rice Pudding with Sour Cherries

This recipe is wonderful for kids, giving them long-lasting carbohydrates, fruit, and milk. Its creamy sweetness blended with fall spices makes grownups love it, too!

INGREDIENTS | SERVES 6

Nonstick spray, as needed

2 cups basmati rice, cooked

1½ cups 2% milk

2 eggs

1 teaspoon vanilla

1 teaspoon salt

¼ cup sugar substitute

¼ teaspoon nutmeg

¼ teaspoon mace

1 cup sour pie cherries, drained, not in sugar syrup

1 tablespoon butter, soft

1. Preheat oven to 325°F. Spray a 2-quart baking dish with nonstick spray. Add the rice.

2. Whisk together the milk, eggs, vanilla, salt, sugar substitute, nutmeg, and mace. Stir in cherries and butter. Mix into the rice.

3. Bake for 50 minutes. Serve warm or chilled.

> **TIP:** *Substitute heart-healthy margarine for butter and replace 2% milk with nonfat milk.*

PER SERVING: Calories: 165 | GI: Low | Carbohydrates: 26g | Protein: 6g | Fat: 5g

Sugar Substitutes

You can use a sugar substitute, such as Splenda, in almost any dessert recipe to lower its GI. The exceptions are in desserts that require caramelizing sugar. (These include flan and brittle.) Just follow directions but remember that substitutes are actually sweeter than sugar.

Whipped Cream

The best whipped cream does not come out of an aerosol can!
Try making it yourself to create a rich, creamy topping for a variety of desserts.

**INGREDIENTS | 1 CUP WHIPPED CREAM,
4 SERVINGS**

½ cup whipping or heavy cream
1 teaspoon sugar substitute, or to taste
Optional: 1 teaspoon vanilla extract

Vanilla

Vanilla is the second-most expensive spice in the world next to saffron. Vanilla beans are the fruit of an orchid plant that originated in Mexican tropical forests and are now cultivated in tropical areas near the Indian Ocean and the South Pacific. Vanilla extract is made from soaking chopped vanilla beans in an alcohol-based solution for several months. Due to the high price of vanilla, many vanilla extracts are made from synthetic vanilla. To avoid imitation vanilla, read the label to make sure it contains "pure" vanilla.

Using an electric mixer or wire whisk (not a blender or food processor), beat the cream on medium-low, adding the sugar substitute a bit at a time. Add vanilla. Don't overbeat, or you'll make butter!

PER SERVING: Calories: 90 | GI: Very low | Carbohydrates: 0g | Protein: 0g | Fat: 9g

Old-Fashioned Apple and Peach Crisp

This is a perfect end-of-summer dish. The apples are just ripening, and the peaches are on their way out. Combining the two is wonderful! You can serve warm or chilled, plain, with whipped cream, or with ice cream!

INGREDIENTS | SERVES 4

Nonstick spray, as needed

2 tart apples, peeled, cored, and sliced

4 medium peaches, blanched, skins and pits removed, sliced

Juice of ½ lemon

½ cup flour

¼ cup dark brown sugar

½ teaspoon cinnamon

½ teaspoon salt

½ teaspoon coriander seed, ground

½ teaspoon cardamom seed, ground

1 cup oatmeal

½ stick butter, softened

1. Preheat the oven to 350°F. Prepare a gratin dish or baking dish with nonstick spray.

2. Distribute the apple and peach slices in the dish and sprinkle with lemon juice.

3. Using your hands, thoroughly mix together the flour, brown sugar, spices, oatmeal, and butter. Spread over the crisp and bake for 45 minutes, or until the fruit is bubbling and the top is brown. Serve with vanilla ice cream or whipped cream.

> **TIP:** *Substitute low-fat frozen yogurt for ice cream or whipped cream to make this a healthier dessert. You could also replace the butter with heart-healthy margarine.*

PER SERVING: Calories: 360 | GI: Moderate | Carbohydrates: 60g | Protein: 6g | Fat: 14g

Baked Apples Stuffed with Nuts and Raisins

For breakfast or dessert, baked apples are a delightful, spicy, and warm treat.

INGREDIENTS | SERVES 2

2 large apples, such as Macintosh, Rome, or Granny Smith

2 teaspoons brown sugar

½ teaspoon cinnamon

2 teaspoons chopped walnuts

2 teaspoons raisins

2 teaspoons butter

2 tablespoons water

Creamy Additions

The spices in these baked, stuffed apples and the tartness of the apples are both complemented nicely by dairy. You can serve these with a little cream poured over the top or a scoop of vanilla ice cream on the side for added richness.

1. Preheat the oven to 350°F. Using a corer, remove the center portions of the apples, being careful not to cut through the bottom of the apple.

2. For each apple, form a cup with a double layer of aluminum foil, going ⅓ of the way up the apple. This will stabilize the apple when baking.

3. Mix together the brown sugar, cinnamon, walnuts, and raisins and stuff the mixture into the apples. Top each apple with 1 teaspoon butter. Put 1 tablespoon water into each aluminum foil cup.

4. Bake for 25 minutes, or until the apples are soft when pricked with a fork.

TIP: *Replace butter with heart-healthy margarine.*

PER SERVING: Calories: 181 | GI: Low | Carbohydrates: 28g | Protein: 1g | Fat: 8g

Grilled Nectarines with Mascarpone and Raspberry Granita

The combination of mascarpone cheese, which is a rich, triple-cream cow's milk cheese, and the sweetness of the nectarines is sublime. Grilling the nectarines brings out their juicy flavor.

INGREDIENTS | SERVES 2

2 nectarines, cut in halves, pits discarded

4 teaspoons mascarpone cheese

4 tablespoons Raspberry Granita (see Chapter 16)

Optional: fresh raspberries for garnish

1. Place the nectarines cut-side down on a hot grill for 5 minutes.

2. Spoon the mascarpone into the depressions left by the pits. Add raspberry granita and serve immediately. If you like, top each nectarine half with a fresh raspberry.

PER SERVING: Calories: 108 | GI: Low | Carbohydrates: 16g | Protein: 2g | Fat: 5g

Frosted Blueberries with Peach Ice

This is an icy treat on a hot day, and they are great at night, too!

INGREDIENTS | SERVES 4

1 cup fresh blueberries

1 tablespoon confectioners' sugar

4 fresh peaches, blanched, halved, pitted, and skins removed

Juice of ½ lemon

½ cup sugar substitute

1½ cups water

1. Cover a baking sheet with aluminum foil. Rinse blueberries and place them while still damp on the sheet and freeze. After 2 hours, sprinkle with confectioners' sugar, roll to coat, cover with plastic wrap, and return to the freezer.

2. Place the peaches, lemon juice, sugar substitute, and water in the blender and purée until very smooth.

3. Pour the peach mixture into an ice cube tray and freeze for 2 hours. Remove and break up with a fork. Continue to freeze until you have a very grainy, icy mixture.

4. Fold the peach slush and blueberries together. Serve in wine goblets.

PER SERVING: Calories: 70 | GI: Low | Carbohydrates: 24g | Protein: 1g | Fat: 0g

Raspberry Granita

Nothing tastes fresher than the pure fruit ice in this recipe!

INGREDIENTS | SERVES 4

1 quart raspberries

1 cup water

4 packets sugar substitute

1 tablespoon lemon juice

Pinch salt

Champagne and Granité

Granita is a sweetened, often fruit-flavored ice with a granular texture. For this recipe, add a splash of Champagne to the mixture before freezing to make an elegant dessert for entertaining.

1. Bring all ingredients to a boil in a medium saucepan.

2. Reduce heat and simmer, covered, for 10 minutes, or until the sugar substitute melts.

3. Force the mixture through a sieve and freeze, breaking up with a fork occasionally. Continue to freeze and break apart until you have a very grainy, icy mixture.

PER SERVING: Calories: 61 | GI: Low | Carbohydrates: 7g | Protein: 1g | Fat: 1g

Nut-Crusted Key Lime Pie

Nut crusts are versatile and very good with almost any kind of pie. Although nuts are fattening, they are still good for you—they contain high amounts of fiber and vitamin E.

INGREDIENTS | SERVES 8

1 cup macadamia nuts, pecans, or walnuts, coarsely ground

1 cup graham cracker crumbs

1 stick butter, melted

1 tablespoon dark brown sugar

Rind of ½ orange

Nonstick spray, as needed

1½ cups cold water

⅓ cup cornstarch

Juice of 3 limes

2 packets unflavored gelatin

2 egg yolks

3 egg whites, beaten stiff

2 tablespoons sugar substitute

1. In the food processor or blender, mix the nuts, cracker crumbs, butter, brown sugar, and orange rind to the texture of oatmeal.

2. Prepare a 9" pie pan with nonstick spray and press the nut mixture into it. Bake in a 325°F oven for 30 minutes, or until crisp and lightly browned. Set aside to cool, then refrigerate.

3. In the blender, mix 1 cup water and all remaining ingredients but the egg whites and sugar substitute. Add the rest of the water and pour into a saucepan. Whisking constantly, bring to a boil. Cool until almost stiff.

4. Place the lime mixture in the well-chilled pie shell. Fold the sugar into the beaten egg whites and spread over lime filling.

5. Place pie in the oven to bake at 350°F until golden brown.

PER SERVING (1" PIECE): Calories: 348 | GI: Crust–low; filling–zero | Carbohydrates: 68g | Protein: 6g | Fat: 27g

Meringue Piecrust

Any number of fillings are wonderful in this piecrust. It should be used the same day you make it. Once filled or sitting out in a humid room, it will turn soggy.

INGREDIENTS | MAKES A 9" PIECRUST

Nonstick spray, as needed

4 egg whites

Pinch salt

1 teaspoon vinegar

½ cup sugar substitute, or to taste

½ cup toasted walnuts, hazelnuts, or pecans

1. Prepare a 9" pie pan with nonstick spray. Beat egg whites by adding salt and then vinegar and sugar substitute. When stiff, fold in nuts.

2. Pile into pie pan. Bake at 175°F for 3–4 hours.

3. Let cool before filling.

PER SERVING (8 SLICES): Calories: 100 | GI: Zero | Carbohydrates: 6g | Protein: 4g | Fat: 9g

Fruit and Cream Filling for Meringue Piecrust

This is the classic filling for Pavlova cake, a wonderful Australian dessert. The cake is sometimes topped with peeled, sliced kiwi fruit in addition to strawberries, which you could do for this recipe as well.

INGREDIENTS | SERVES 8

1 Meringue Piecrust (see pervious recipe)

1 banana

1 cup heavy or whipping cream

2 teaspoons sugar substitute, plus 1 tablespoon

1 teaspoon vanilla extract

1 pint strawberries, washed and hulled; half sliced, half left whole for top of pie

1. Using a cool Meringue Piecrust, slice the banana over the bottom of the crust.

2. Whip the cream with 2 teaspoons sugar substitute and vanilla. Spoon and spread on half the whipped cream mixture.

3. Cover with the sliced strawberries; sprinkle with remaining sugar substitute.

4. Cover with whipped cream and arrange the rest of the berries on top. Serve immediately.

PER SERVING (CRUST NOT INCLUDED): Calories: 116 | GI: Very low | Carbohydrates: 6g | Protein: 0g | Fat: 9g

Raspberry or Strawberry Coulis

This is delectable over ice cream, sherbet, or sorbet.

INGREDIENTS | **MAKES 6 OUNCES (6 SERVINGS)**

8 ounces strawberries or raspberries, washed and hulled

1 teaspoon lemon juice

Sugar substitute, to taste (start with 1 packet)

Blend all ingredients in the blender. Strain and serve.

PER SERVING: Calories: 8 | GI: Very low | Carbohydrates: 2g | Protein: 0g | Fat: 0g

Flourless Hazelnut Chocolate Cake

In this melt-in-your-mouth cake, nutrient-dense high glycemic index white flour
is replaced by nutrient-dense hazelnuts.

INGREDIENTS | SERVES 12

Nonstick spray, as needed

3½ cups ground roasted hazelnuts

1½ cups Splenda No Calorie Sweetener, granulated

2 tablespoons vanilla extract

¾ cup unsweetened cocoa

12 egg whites

1. Preheat oven to 350°F. Coat a 10" springform pan with nonstick cooking spray.

2. Mix hazelnuts, Splenda, vanilla, and cocoa in a medium-sized bowl. Beat egg whites until stiff. Gently fold the egg whites into the chocolate nut mixture.

3. Pour batter into greased pan. Bake 40–50 minutes or until toothpick inserted into cake comes out clean.

4. Cool before serving.

PER SERVING: Calories: 334 | GI: Low | Carbohydrates: 34g | Protein: 9g | Fat: 20g

Coconut Macaroons

A light and fluffy flourless dessert. It's difficult to have just one!

INGREDIENTS | MAKES 20 SERVINGS

6 egg whites

Pinch salt

⅓ cup agave nectar

1 teaspoon vanilla extract

¼ teaspoon almond extract

3 cups unsweetened coconut, shredded

1. Preheat oven to 350°F. Using an electric mixer, beat egg whites and salt until stiff.

2. In a second bowl, combine agave nectar, vanilla, and almond extract. Using a folding motion, combine coconut and agave mixture with egg whites.

3. Place tablespoon-sized portions of coconut batter onto a baking sheet lined with parchment paper. Using fingers, mold macaroons into a round shape.

4. Bake for 15 minutes, until slightly golden brown.

PER SERVING: Calories: 100 | GI: Zero | Carbohydrates: 4g | Protein: 2g | Fat: 9g

Dark Chocolate–Dipped Macaroons

A favorite for chocolate lovers, dark chocolate is both tasty and has a low glycemic value.

INGREDIENTS | MAKES 20 SERVINGS

2 cups water

4 ounces dark chocolate chips

1 batch Coconut Macaroons (see previous recipe)

1. Add water to the bottom of a double boiler. Bring water to a simmer and turn heat down to low. Add chocolate to the pan and stir with a wooden spoon until melted.

2. Dip macaroons halfway into the chocolate to coat. Place dipped macaroons onto a tray covered with parchment paper.

3. Place tray of macaroons in the refrigerator to allow chocolate to harden.

PER SERVING: Calories: 133 | GI: Very low | Carbohydrates: 6g | Protein: 2g | Fat: 11g

Almond Cookies

Rich in healthy fats and vitamin E, almonds are known for promoting heart health.

INGREDIENTS | SERVES 12

2 cups almonds
¼ cup pecans
½ teaspoon salt
⅓ cup rolled oats
⅓ cup flaxseed, ground
1 teaspoon baking powder
1 teaspoon vanilla extract
1 teaspoon cinnamon
3 tablespoons butter, softened
⅔ cup agave nectar
Nonstick spray, as needed

1. Chop almonds and pecans; set aside 3 tablespoons almonds. Lightly toast the nuts in the oven. Place nuts in a food processor and grind until a butter-like consistency forms.

2. Add all the ingredients except the agave nectar and process. Finally, add the agave nectar to the dough and process until incorporated.

3. Spray a cookie sheet with nonstick cooking spray or line with parchment paper. Make dough into 1" balls, place on cookie sheet, and flatten down. Sprinkle with reserved chopped almonds.

4. Bake at 350°F for 10 minutes, until just slightly browned.

PER SERVING: Calories: 171 | GI: Very low | Carbohydrates: 8g | Protein: 5g | Fat: 14g

Berry Crumble

Try this recipe with a variety of succulent berries to satisfy your sweet tooth.

INGREDIENTS | SERVES 4

1 12-ounce bag frozen berries, or 2 cups fresh berries

4 tablespoons unsalted butter, softened

3 tablespoons Splenda No Calorie Sweetener, granulated

2 large eggs

1 teaspoon vanilla extract

¼ teaspoon salt

½ teaspoon baking powder

½ cup almond flour

1. Place berries in an 8" × 8" glass baking dish.

2. In a medium mixing bowl, whip butter and Splenda with a fork. Mix in eggs, vanilla, and salt until well blended.

3. In a separate bowl, stir together the baking powder and almond flour. Add almond flour mixture to the butter and egg mixture and mix well.

4. Spread the batter over the fruit. Bake at 375°F for 25 minutes, until golden brown on top.

PER SERVING: Calories: 211 | GI: Very low | Carbohydrates: 11g | Protein: 7g | Fat: 21g

Cinnamon Nut Cookies

The base of this cookie is whole-wheat flour and walnuts.
It is tasty and at the same time healthy enough to be eaten for breakfast!

INGREDIENTS | SERVES 24

2 cups walnuts

1 cup whole-wheat flour

½ cup almond flour

¼ cup flaxseed, ground

1 teaspoon cinnamon

¼ teaspoon salt

¾ cup Splenda No Calorie Sweetener, granulated

¾ cup butter, softened

1 large egg

1. Preheat oven to 300°F.

2. Add walnuts, flours, flaxseeds, cinnamon, and salt to food processor. Process until the nuts are finely chopped.

3. In a medium mixing bowl, add the Splenda to the softened butter and beat to combine; add the egg and mix well. Mix the dry ingredients into the butter mixture until well combined.

4. Place tablespoon-sized pieces of dough on ungreased cookie sheets. Press cookies to flatten and make cookie shape, spacing them 1½"–2" apart.

5. Bake for 15 minutes until slightly browned.

PER SERVING: Calories: 151 | GI: Very low | Carbohydrates: 6g | Protein: 3g | Fat: 14g

Grilled Peaches Filled with Mascarpone Cheese and Rosemary

You may serve this as a savory brunch dish, or mix the mascarpone with some sugar for a dessert.

INGREDIENTS | SERVES 2

2 ripe peaches, split, pits removed

4 teaspoons mascarpone cheese, at room temperature

1 teaspoon fresh rosemary, chopped

Salt and pepper, to taste

1. Place the peaches cut-side down on a hot grill until they soften, about 4 minutes.

2. Mix the cheese, rosemary, salt, and pepper.

3. Turn peaches and stuff with cheese filling. Grill for 2–3 minutes.

PER SERVING: Calories: 61 | GI: Very low | Carbohydrates: 7g | Protein: 46g | Fat: 3g

Chocolate-Dipped Fruit

This fondue-style treat melts in your mouth.

INGREDIENTS | SERVES 3

6 large strawberries

1 pear

1 underripe banana

3 cups water

⅓ cup dark chocolate chips

1. Wash fruit and peel banana. Slice banana into 1"-thick pieces. Core pear and slice into 6 pieces.

2. Add water to the bottom of a double boiler. Bring water to a simmer and turn heat down to low. Add chocolate to the double boiler and stir with a wooden spoon until melted.

3. Using fingers or a skewer, dip fruit pieces halfway into the chocolate to coat. Place dipped fruit onto a tray covered with parchment paper.

4. Place the tray in the refrigerator to allow chocolate to harden. Results are best if served the same day.

PER SERVING: Calories: 189 | GI: Low | Carbohydrates: 31g | Protein: 2g | Fat: 7g

Strawberry-Rhubarb Pudding

This is a wonderful flavor for spring. It's low in fat and carbohydrates, and has a low GI.

INGREDIENTS | SERVES 4

1 envelope unflavored gelatin

¼ cup cold water

1 cup fresh rhubarb, cut into 1" pieces

¼ cup water

½ pint strawberries, washed, hulled, and sliced (half reserved for topping)

½ cup Splenda No Calorie Sweetener, granulated

2 cups nonfat vanilla yogurt

1. Place the gelatin in the cold water in the jar of a blender.

2. In a saucepan over medium heat, boil the rhubarb, ¼ cup water, and half the strawberries with the Splenda.

3. Add the hot fruit to the gelatin and pulse to chop and mix the gelatin with the fruit. Cool to room temperature.

4. Swirl the fruit and yogurt together and spoon into glasses or bowls. Add strawberries for topping.

PER SERVING: Calories: 195 | GI: Very low | Carbohydrates: 41g | Protein: 10g | Fat: 0g

Additional Information

THE DIABETES NETWORK

This website is useful for looking up information about the GI, as well as for determining the GI value of specific foods.
www.diabetesnet.com

THE GLUTEN-FREE MALL

This is a fine source for all kinds of rice and a variety of flours. Whether you are worried about gluten or not, it's a resource for many products that may be hard to find in your local stores.
www.GlutenFreeMall.com

IRISH OATMEAL

McCann's and Flavahan's are two brands of Irish oatmeal, which is cut more coarsely than quick oats for maximum advantage to low GI diets. These brands are available nationally in all major food chains.

NATIONAL DIABETES INFORMATION CLEARINGHOUSE (NDIC)

NDIC is a service of the National Institute of Diabetes and Digestive and Kidney Diseases, a part of the National Institutes of Health. The mission of NDIC is to increase knowledge and understanding about diabetes among patients, health care providers, and the public.
http://diabetes.niddk.nih.gov/index.htm

SPLENDA, NO CALORIE SWEETENER, GRANULATED

This is an excellent sugar substitute for use in custards, pie fillings, cheesecakes, puddings, sweet sauces, frostings, homemade ice cream, and sorbets. It's not recommended when you want to brown a cookie or cake or caramelize a topping. Then, Splenda Sugar Blend is excellent—it has half the calories of sugar and provides enough sugar for texture and browning. Bakers like it because it holds up well—it doesn't break down or get bitter when exposed to heat.
www.splenda.com

TRADER JOE'S

A national chain, Trader Joe's has some of the most interesting foods available. Their frozen foods and other private-label products are excellent, and their nuts are a bargain.
www.traderjoes.com

WILD OATS

Wild Oats is a chain of natural food stores specializing in organic fresh, frozen, dried, and prepared foods. They have many whole-grain and low GI products from breads and cereals to cookies and cakes.

Glycemic Index Reference Books

Brand-Miller, Jennie, Joanna McMillan-Price, and Kaye Foster-Powell. *The Low GI Diet Revolution*. New York: Marlowe & Co., 2005.

Brand-Miller, Jennie, and Kaye Foster-Powell. *The New Glucose Revolution Shopper's Guide to GI Values 2010: The Authoritative Source of Glycemic Index Values for More Than 1,300 Foods*. Cambridge, MA: Da Capo Press, 2010.

Brand-Miller, Jennie, Kaye Foster-Powell, Stephen Colagiuri, and Alan Barclay. *The New Glucose Revolution for Diabetes: The Definitive Guide to Managing Diabetes and Prediabetes Using the Glycemic Index*. New York: Marlowe & Co., 2007.

Brand-Miller, Jennie, Kaye Foster-Powell, Stephen Colagiuri, and Thomas M.S. Wolever. *The Glucose Revolution Pocket Guide to Diabetes*. New York: Marlowe & Co., 2001.

Brand-Miller, Jennie, Kaye Foster-Powell, Stephen Colagiuri, and Thomas M. S. Wolever. *The Glucose Revolution Pocket Guide to Sports Nutrition*. New York: Marlowe & Co., 2001.

Brand-Miller, Jennie, Kaye Foster-Powell, Stephen Colagiuri, and Thomas M. S. Wolever. *The Glucose Revolution Pocket Guide to Your Heart*. New York: Marlowe & Co., 2001.

Brand-Miller, Jennie, Kaye Foster-Powell, Stephen Colagiuri, and Thomas M. S. Wolever. *The New Glucose Revolution*. New York: Marlowe & Co., 1996, 2003, 2005.

Cunningham, Marion. *The Fannie Farmer Cookbook, 13th Edition*. New York: Alfred Knopf, 1996.

Gallop, Rick. *The G.I. Diet*. New York: Workman Publishing, 2010.

Woodruff, Sandra. *The Good Carb Cookbook*. New York: Avery Press, 2001.

Index

We Have
EVERYTHING
on Anything!

The Everything® list spans a wide range of subjects, with more than 500 titles covering 25 different categories:

Business	History	Reference
Careers	Home Improvement	Religion
Children's Storybooks	Everything Kids	Self-Help
Computers	Languages	Sports & Fitness
Cooking	Music	Travel
Crafts and Hobbies	New Age	Wedding
Education/Schools	Parenting	Writing
Games and Puzzles	Personal Finance	
Health	Pets	